Banning Queer Blood

Banning Queer Blood

Rhetorics of Citizenship,
Contagion, and Resistance

Jeffrey A. Bennett

The University of Alabama Press
Tuscaloosa

Copyright © 2009
The University of Alabama Press
Tuscaloosa, Alabama 35487-0380
All rights reserved
Manufactured in the United States of America

Typeface: Bembo

∞

The paper on which this book is printed meets the minimum requirements of
American National Standard for Information Sciences-Permanence of Paper for
Printed Library Materials, ANSI Z39.48-1984.

Library of Congress Cataloging-in-Publication Data

Bennett, Jeffrey A. (Jeffrey Allen), 1974–
    Banning queer blood : rhetorics of citizenship, contagion, and resistance /
Jeffrey A. Bennett.
        p. ; cm. — (Rhetoric, culture, and social critique)
    Includes bibliographical references and index.
    ISBN 978-0-8173-1664-8 (cloth : alk. paper) 1. Blood donors. 2. Gay men.
3. Blood—Collection and preservation—Social aspects. I. Title. II. Series: Rhetoric,
culture, and social critique.
    [DNLM: 1. Blood Donors. 2. Homosexuality, Male. 3. Health Policy. 4. Social
Identification. 5. Social Responsibility. WH 460 B471b 2009]
    RM172.B46 2009
    362.17'8408664—dc22

                                                                      2009005077

For my mother, Sandra
and my father, Allen

Contents

Acknowledgments

In the weeks after I completed an initial draft of this manuscript I was diagnosed a type-one diabetic. The depressing irony of writing for years about the constitution of contaminated blood and then being informed my own blood was, in fact, deficient, seemed a tad unusual, if not cruel. Suddenly, the ways blood structures everyday life and long-term health was something I contemplated and confronted constantly. Although a painful way to learn about the import of blood, my experiences with diabetes have allowed me to ponder the symbolic and material consequences of blood in ways unimaginable years ago. I am more aware than ever that the sanguine substance is intimately tied to both identity and public culture. Blood is a metaphor of life and of death; it fosters insider and outsider relations; it has economic clout and emblematic significance; it is a gift, a sacrifice, a commodity, and a taboo. Indeed, the meanings we bring to this primal fluid are far from natural, organic, or self-evident, being imbued with cultural connotations reflecting imagined connectedness, tentative securities, and demonstrable anxieties. For example, several times daily, when my blood is tested, glucose meters attempt to numerically signify something happening in my body that is unstable and prone to sudden change. These numbers gauge not only the degree to which my blood is "normal," they also speak to issues of control, excess, demise, judgment, technologies of health, and the management of the body. These constructs, in both the blood ban and diabetes, guide approaches to blood regulation that have serious implications on public conversations grappling with the ramifications of freedom and restraint.

Nonetheless, for many people blood inspires alarm and revulsion because of the abject discomfort it projects. Images of blood are often censored in news stories about war, the production of food, and the birth of children. People regularly flinch with unease at the sight of my finger being pricked in public spaces for premeal testing. However, we are also fascinated with and deferential to blood, representing it on artifacts such as the U.S. flag and symbolically drinking the blood of deities each Sunday. The undercurrents of blood structure various aspects of the polis and are ever present if you simply look close enough. These economic, cultural, personal, and rhetorical issues speak volumes about the ways blood functions publicly and the effect it can have on each of us, especially those most implicated in blood policies and their stigmatizing force.

Thankfully, writing a book underscored by references to kinship and group-belonging also magnifies beneficial relations among people, not simply the maniacal workings of state agencies. This book has profited from hours of conversation with good friends about blood donation and the insinuations prompted by bureaucratic exclusion. I would like to express gratitude for the many talks I have had with friends over meals, coffee, and drinks, including Cara Buckley, Tonia Edwards, Paula Figard, Shane Grant, Claire King, Matt King, Dawn Knox, Karen Kostrinsky, John Lynch, Scott Makstenieks, Tom Mentzer, Leigh Moscowitz, Jeff Motter, Bill and Pam Newberry, Kate Hess Pace, Jamie Skerski, Sue Stanfield, Frank Reynolds, Brenda Walleman, Kerith Woodyard, and Patricia Young. I am especially grateful to those friends who read and enhanced chapters with their generous and insightful feedback, including Darrel Enck-Wanzer, Suzanne Enck-Wanzer, Melanie Loehwing, and David Moscowitz.

My colleagues at Georgia State University have conveyed much enthusiasm for the project and I appreciate their continued support. I am especially indebted to David Cheshier, James Darsey, Alisa Perren, Alessandra Raengo, Angelo Restivo, Mary Stuckey, and Holley Wilkin. Mary read every chapter of the book and her thoughtful comments are reflected in its final form. This study also benefited from the labor, feedback, and research assistance of Kimberly Huff and Laurel Berryman. Professionally, I appreciate the backing this book has received in various forms from Carol Greenhouse, Larry Gross, Charles Morris, Tom Nakayama, and Gust Yep.

The faculty at Indiana University, whom I count as dear friends, helped create a space in rhetorical studies where the work I do is regarded not as "identity politics," but as progressive cultural critique. To name just a few, this study profited from Robert Terrill's close readings of the text and his infectious humor. Tom Foster introduced me to queer theory, providing an essential foundation to this work. Phaedra Pezzullo provided amazing support, eagerly helping with everything from the content of the text to the cover it dons. John Lucaites has long expressed excitement for the project and years later he continues to affirm this venture with equal exhilaration. Perhaps more than any other, Robert Ivie's guidance permeates this volume. His friendship, advice, and mentorship have left a special imprint on my thought. His insights regarding scapegoating, symbolism, and criticism radiate from this book.

The men who pass to donate blood and protest at the ritual site deserve special mention. Their passion for equality and their insights regarding donation privileges made the fifth chapter a delight to write. I am appreciative for their time, their voices, and their sacrifices. I hope readers learn as much as I have from their creative transgressions.

Conversely, numerous blood agencies provided valuable research information. I want to thank various representatives from local chapters of the American Red Cross, the American Association of Blood Banks, America's Blood Centers, the Food and Drug Administration, Canadian Blood Services, and the National Marrow Donor Program for information they imparted to make this a more accurate and compelling project.

A special thanks to the editors and staff at the University of Alabama Press who have been supportive throughout this process.

Portions of chapter 5 were originally published under the title "Passing, Protesting, and the Arts of Resistance: Infiltrating the Ritual Space of Blood Donation" in the *Quarterly Journal of Speech* 94, 1 (February 2008): 23–43. Thanks to Taylor and Francis (http://www.tandf.co.uk) for allowing me to reprint my work here.

If kinship is a central part of this text it may be attributed to my extensive expertise in the subject. My extended family counts no fewer than eighteen aunts, sixteen uncles, and forty cousins. While there is little room to thank all of them, I want to mention especially my grandparents, Lorraine and Richard Danford, Carol and Harold Bennett, and Zelma Reece. I am fortunate to have siblings that I count as close friends and allies. So, I thank my brothers, sisters, and sisters-in-law for their love and support: Scott, Barb, Randy, Sharon, Katie, Michael, James, and Katie. And for the hope they give me, I thank Brianna, Scotty, Tyler, and Brayden.

My parents, Sandra and Scott Lewis and Allen and Kathy Bennett, have long stressed the importance of ideas and the inherent goodness in people. My mother and father have been good friends, engaging conversationalists, and wonderful human beings. As great parents are prone to do, they have always grown with me as much as I have grown with them.

Finally, I would be lost without my partner, Isaac West. His spirit, honesty, and care are as ubiquitous in this project as they are in my life. He was there when diabetes imposed itself on me and will assuredly be there when it departs. My world is made brighter by his love, his encouragement, and, most especially, his laughter.

1
Queer Citizenship and the Stigma of Banned Blood

In the days following the attacks on the World Trade Center on September 11, 2001, the late Reverend Jerry Falwell took to the airwaves to explain where America had gone wrong. Appearing on Pat Robertson's *The 700 Club*, Falwell employed a predictable and tired jeremiad, alleging that America's tolerance of secular values, promoted primarily by feminists and gay rights advocates, invited the assaults. Without hesitation he incriminated his usual suspects, asserting, "I point the finger in their face and say, 'you helped this happen.'"[1] Falwell's hyperbolic and opportunistic remarks provoked a wellspring of criticism from a variety of state officials, lobbying groups, and grieving citizens. He was chastised by conservatives and liberals alike for trivializing the rationale of terrorists and implicating gays and lesbians in such a ridiculous plot.[2]

As Falwell was scolded for his prejudice and poor political timing, people across the country ascribed meaning to the week's events. Extraordinary acts of national unity transpired as citizens held vigils, lit candles, raised flags, and supported local blood drives. The act of donating blood seemed to carry especially significant cultural capital. By the end of the day on September 11, the American Red Cross (ARC) blood donation telephone line received more than a million calls from citizens eager to help with relief efforts, breaking the previous record of three thousand calls in one day. The next morning, at the request of President George Bush's staff, a blood drive was held in the White House. Keeping to form, Congress initiated a two-day blood drive for offices in the House of Representatives and the Senate. In fact, in "the first month following the attacks alone, the Red Cross collected 2 million units of blood and more than a quarter of a million donors gave for the first time."[3]

Among those people to show up at churches, schools, town halls, and other institutions of civic importance for the first time were untold numbers of queer men.[4] One by one, as they rolled up their sleeves eager to invoke their support, they were turned away from these quotidian sites of civic performance. Each of these men was told individually that he was a member of a "high risk" group. All of them carried this label regardless of the longevity and monogamy of their relationships, their safe-sex practices, or their desire to be woven into the fabric of our national identity. Like most Americans, these men likely scoffed at Falwell's remarks positioning them as a threat to national security. But unlike most citizens, they also learned that the mentality guiding the media-driven minister is ubiquitous in a cultural discourse that ritualistically forbids queer men from donating blood.

At the height of the AIDS scare in the early 1980s, the Food and Drug Administration (FDA), in conjunction with the Public Health Service (PHS), implemented donor exclusion policies prohibiting blood donations from any man who engaged in sexual activity with another man.[5] At the time, little was known about Acquired Immune Deficiency Syndrome (AIDS) or effective methods of prevention. An unknown number of individuals were contracting HIV from blood transfusions and an unfolding national crisis demanded immediate action. When government agencies issued their public health recommendations in 1983 there was little institutional support for spurring educational initiatives, scant proof that AIDS was caused by a virus, and no scientifically tested methods for recognizing HIV in the blood supply.

Improved testing methods now reliably detect HIV within days of donation. As such, the odds of contracting HIV through blood transfusions are extraordinarily minuscule. Unfortunately, the criteria for determining who should, and should not, contribute blood have not evolved with scientific advancements. Despite medical and technological progress, discriminatory attitudes continue to underwrite the unwarranted policy. Time and again the FDA's Blood Products Advisory Committee (BPAC) has narrowly upheld the long-standing ban on accepting blood donations, *indefinitely,* from any man who has "had sexual contact with another male, *even once,* since 1977."[6] The agency has denied vehemently that this policy is a direct attack on the character and integrity of queer men, asserting that such moves are a matter of public health, not group stigma.[7] Nonetheless, the rejection of this blood illustrates a complex cultural management, a disciplining of citizenship and its affiliation with performances of nationalism. Constructing queer identity through representations of diseased and undisciplined sexuality, the state mobilizes rhetorics consistent with Iris Marion Young's disconcerting observation that queer people are perhaps the most abject Other in the United States.[8]

Advocates of the ban have concocted, deployed, and stubbornly adhered to detrimental constructs of queer men. These constructs frame disturbing judgments, erode legitimate claims to full citizenship, and reproduce preju-

dice rather than epidemiological knowledge. Such attitudes reflect the treacherous terrain on which queers must operate. Indeed, this convoluted discourse,
which denies queer men the opportunity to donate blood to fellow citizens by
negotiating gender and sexuality at the intersection of science, civil society,
and the state, elucidates the very vanishing point of citizenship that queers
confront daily. However, unlike other flash points in the culture wars such as
gay marriage, adoption, or the gays in the military debate, the blood ban operates on the margins of cultural visibility, receiving scant attention from the
popular press and lesbian, gay, bisexual, and transgender (LGBT) lobby organizations. Despite this erasure, its potency to sustain an image of queer men
as dangerous to both local communities and national security should not be
dismissed. Approximately twenty-two thousand people donate blood to the
ARC daily. And every one of them, regardless of sex, race, class, religion,
sexual orientation, and political affiliation confront the question: are you a
"male who has had sexual contact with another male, even once, since 1977?"[9]
While it is impossible to surmise how each citizen reacts to that that inquiry,
it must give pause to many. How does such a question shape understandings
of queer men?[10] And, even more important, how does it simultaneously continue the articulation between queer men and AIDS while disarticulating
their roles as active, informed, and valued citizens?

Imagining the polluted stranger who wanders dangerously within the
polity is not without precedent. Although *Banning Queer Blood* is grounded in
a contemporary American context, it is conversant with an amorphous set of
discourses that have been echoed, albeit differently, throughout history. The
practice of isolating a population and segregating their blood, both literally
and symbolically, is certainly not a new phenomenon. Women, Jews, African
Americans, and any number of cultures around the globe have been positioned as impure threats for centuries. Queer citizens are but another population implicated in disparaging discourses of disciplinary social institutions.
While certain historical contexts set this instance of blood segregation apart
from others, understanding these diabolical stigmas is aided by examining
cognate genealogies. The rhetoric of the blood ban entails unique tropes and
characteristics, but it can also offer significant understandings of how blood
and the body are part of a larger history of segregation, citizenship, and national identity. Notably, the blood-ban debate is not specific to the United
States, but circulates globally in countries as diverse as Malaysia, Canada, Scot-
land, Australia, South Africa, Japan, and Portugal.

The focus on communal identity and sacrificial ritual means that this book
is first and foremost concerned with citizenship: how it is constructed, articulated, performed, and reiterated in all its complexity. If citizenship is the tenor

of this analysis, the blood ban is its vehicle, offering a site for probing the discursive constraints placed on queer identity in American culture. At a time when LGBT rights are garnering an increasing degree of public attention, it is important to explore how stigma stubbornly holds its ground, including the ways matters of "public health" become rhetorically separated from, and ultimately trump, claims to "civil liberties." Ascertaining the cultural investment the state has traditionally had in maintaining discourses of purity, especially as they are intertwined with powerful narratives grounded in science and law, illuminates the role institutions play in the development of epistemological and ontological understandings of queer bodies.

The blood ban magnifies formidable manifestations of the performance of citizenship, signaling a larger political struggle to direct the public transcripts of inclusion and democracy. Public transcripts, James Scott explains, are a shorthand way of describing the open interaction between those who dominate and the people they attempt to subordinate.[11] These sites of discursive contestation negotiate stranger-relationality and lay the foundation of commonsense notions of normality and anomaly. Authorities frequently aim to manipulate these scripts to depict the scope of institutional power for people with limited access to cultural resources. As such, consequential details concerning the state's ability to perpetuate discrimination are often eclipsed. When the state employs science to guide our understandings of civic performance, for example, terms such as "deviance" and "mental illness" can purport to "remove much of the personal stigma from the labels but they can succeed, simultaneously, in marginalizing resistance in the name of science."[12] Queer citizens have fallen victim to such rhetorics because their embodied sexual digressions mar the purity of civic identities promoted by social institutions.

Exploring complex policy formations inflected by public transcripts of purity and danger, however, is not enough. Rather than accept dominant messages, populations often reject, negotiate, and complicate ideological information to their own ends. These hidden transcripts are characterized as taking place "offstage," past the direct observation of those controlling matters of social significance. While hidden transcripts may uphold the norms of the ruling class, the so-called weapons of the weak produced in the minutia of everyday life also have the power to subvert, compromise, or reject dominating discourses. By demarcating the discrepancy between the hidden and public transcripts, or the places where the two conceptually blur, the impact of domination on discursive formations can be critically assessed.[13] If we accept, as Foucault does, that "power comes from below," hidden transcripts can offer insight for undoing the damage created by the deferral measure. The ways people respond to the blood ban—by tactically lying to evade the policies and protesting to verbalize dissent—are equally significant when scrutinizing these policies.[14]

But this text is not simply about queer people. At the end of this book, I hope all readers agree that banning queer blood is counterproductive to the goodwill necessary for sustaining a transformative democratic practice. The volunteer donor pool is but one victim of this constraining measure. Equally vital is the decay of social bonds among strangers who are given distorted caricatures of queer citizens on a daily basis. These policies do real violence to people aspiring to abet others. With a spirit of rhetorical renovation in mind, this book will advocate for a reimagining of cultural politics in the public sphere. This introductory chapter acts as an orientation to the larger project, concerning itself primarily with the history of blood donation and its relationship to the production of national identifications. The ritual of donating blood is a powerful cultural and rhetorical force that encourages the normalization of civic identity through purified understandings of public sacrifice. This conformity is sustained through medical and legal discourses that divide issues of "public health" from notions of "civil rights," all the while dismissing powerful social, institutional, and economic considerations.

CONSTITUTING CITIZENSHIP: THE PERFORMATIVE ACT OF BLOOD DONATION

The act of donating blood as an altruistic form of civic engagement came to fruition in the throes of the Second World War. As blood transfusion science became increasingly sophisticated, American military forces translated medical miracles into battlefield advantages. New methods for gathering, transporting, storing, and preserving blood saved countless lives. As a point of comparison, during World War I between eight and eleven of every one hundred soldiers who reached a hospital died. By World War II increasingly reliable blood technology dropped the number of casualties to fewer than five of every one hundred men. And by the time of the Korean War the amount was again halved.[15]

While the Allies capitalized on their understanding of blood collection during World War II, countries like Germany technologically and pragmatically disadvantaged themselves. From a scientific standpoint, the Germans were deficient because they had interned a number of their top doctors who had been making progress in blood science. Additionally, while the United States and Britain had adopted methods of collecting blood from citizens for storage, the German army, with a limited understanding of such practices, was completely dependent on the "hoof donor." This meant that donors had to be present in hospitals for direct transfusions to transpire. As a result, countless Allied troops were saved, while German forces suffered dramatically. In addition to medical weaknesses, the Germans were victims of their own prejudices. Their obsession with blood purity led government officials to restrict who was allowed to give blood to soldiers, narrowly constraining donor pools to "Aryans." Not only did the Germans need to get bodies into hospitals for transfusions, they had to locate and then transport a *specific kind* of person to emergency sites.[16]

Blood donation proved to be a valuable ritual for citizens to make a direct contribution to the war effort and lay an individual claim to the defeat of the Axis powers. Extensive campaigns were launched by the government to encourage people to give the gift of life. Being a donor quickly became synonymous with being an actively engaged citizen and a person who supported troops overseas. While blood had always had a close symbolic relationship to kinship, blood donation provided an even more intimate link between citizenship and the community. Giving blood was a simple act that took little time and almost no effort on the part of the donor. Health officials initiated blood drives across the country in locations traditionally associated with civic identity, including churches, schools, hospitals, and town halls.

What is often underscored, and what needs to be made most present here, is the idea that blood donation became a *performative* act of civic engagement and nation building. It was ritualistically incorporated into the national fabric of American life during times of global and local crises. Blood is a biological material with a relatively short life span. It expires quickly, leaving the national supply in constant need of replenishment. Because there is no known substitute for blood, citizens were, and continue to be, regularly solicited to donate and repeat acts of selflessness to help others survive. This altruism performs a connectedness between the citizen and the persons they assume to be helping. In the ritual of blood donation, the individual body functions as a medium of culture, always acting as a representation of a larger social form—that of an engaged citizen.[17]

The performative act of blood donation illuminates the manner in which civic rituals constitute and sustain "truths" that stabilize normative political identities. Cultural theorists such as Judith Butler have famously advanced the performativity of identity to explore issues of gender and sexuality and the ways identities become discursively and materially normalized. The conceptual illusions of continuity addressed by such perspectives provide a productive lens for examining the self-evident cultural norms concerning identity and citizenship in the rhetoric of the blood ban.[18] Far from a simple form of self-expression, the performativity of identity stresses an ambiguous reiterative power of discourse to produce and control subjects. The mimetic force of blood donation acts as a method of recasting national identifications and making communal bonds appear natural. For example, the perpetual blood shortages that regularly necessitate replenishing encourage the repetition of a donor pool that sees itself as providing an important public service that will reinvigorate the supply, enhance community life, and substantiate their ability to be active citizens. The repeated giving of blood is constructed as an inherent virtue whose benefits far exceed its costs. In this performance of citizenship the positive associations of blood donation are symbolically transfused into the moral worth of the blood donor.

It is in the ritual of blood donation that actors come to feel closer to the social body. Like other rites of belonging, blood donation offers "the perception that these practices are distinct and the associations that they engender are special."[19] People do not simply think of blood donation and come to identify themselves as citizens. Rather, it is the act itself that allows people to position themselves as actively engaged, as a functioning part of the social body. Catherine Bell explains, rituals function "as practices that act upon the actions of others, as the mute interplay of complex strategies within a field structured by engagements of power, as the arena for prescribed sequences of repetitive movements of the body that simultaneously constitute the body, the person, and the macro- and micronetworks of power."[20] More than a simple form of altruism, blood donation is a constitutive ritual that produces citizens in the actions it requires.

Citizenship itself is an essentially contested concept and there is no universal agreement about its social utility, political expediency, or ethical merits.[21] Discussions of citizenship take on diffuse permutations depending on the emphasis given to the term (political, economic, social, cultural), the philosophical foundations privileged (ancient Greece, seventeenth-century Enlightenment), and its ideological situatedness (neoliberalism, radical democracy). Some, such as J.G.A. Pocock, embrace the performative nature of citizenship, arguing it "is not just a means to being free; it is the way of being free itself."[22] Others, such as Louis Althusser, more pessimistically contend the "category of the citizen realizes the *synthesis of the State* in man himself: the citizen is the State in the private man."[23] Citizenship's radical indeterminacy does not suggest it has no material or political capital. It simply means citizenship is a fluid concept whose meaning is habitable in particular historical and cultural contexts.

As a fulcrum of meaning production, constituting subjectivities based on broad cultural normativities, incarnations of citizenship act as sites of intelligibility where the materialization of specific rights and obligations come to fruition.[24] The obligations people in a community share typically transcend the legal confirmations of citizenship and ascend into a category of responsibility that is civic, but not wholly dependent on government authority.[25] After all, being a good citizen connotes more than forced service on a jury or in an army. As a signifier forever in process, citizenship is always partial in its constitution of identity. As Toby Miller argues, "Ideal citizenship can never quite be attained, but the drive toward perfection as the best possible consumer, patriot, or ideologue, enjoins the subject to strive for it by the instillation of ethical incompleteness."[26] In short, normativities perpetually mobilize identities, but configurations of citizenship are always incomplete and unstable, inspiring a reproduction of meaning in a polis.[27] Blood donation spikes during national crises because those situations require a reproduction of meaning widely shared among community members. When the exigency subsides, the necessity to fabricate order also recedes.

Despite the enthusiasm citizenship inspires, preoccupation with the concept has produced damaging erasures. The frequent slippage between "people" and "citizens" highlights the marginalization citizenship can foster.[28] Citizenship establishes those who belong from those who do not, defining norms that are often blatantly hostile, intolerant, and xenophobic. The requirements for becoming a citizen, for example, are steeped in cultural connotations that reveal the neuroses (what we often call values) of a state. Any person seeking U.S. citizenship, for example, must renounce allegiance to other states, uphold the Constitution, and know basic political history dictated by public transcripts. People are required to master the fundamentals of speaking, reading, and writing English to establish citizenship. The state also demands individuals to disavow polygamy, not gamble illegally, avoid being a "habitual drunkard," and not support "prostitution or communal vice."[29] While the flexibility regarding public intoxication is no doubt appreciated by many, the strict moral implications of sex are as telling as the donor deferral question lodged at queer men.[30] The citizenship test equates particular forms of sex with espionage and disloyalty, forcing questions about the sanctity of sexual identity and its relation to the state. The reiteration of identity through ritual clarifies who is pure and who is not, sometimes in the shape of a pledge and at other times by way of a blood-donor questionnaire.

Like most rituals that involve national identity and civic performance, blood donation has evolved in a number of ways since the time of World War II. Discourses of purity were recurrently essential to these transformations. These changes transpired over the course of three decades as our understandings of blood and technology progressed. While there is too little room here to discuss all the changes in blood donation that occurred, two points are especially relevant to this project.[31] The first is the development of blood and blood products into a multi-billion-dollar industry. By 1998 the blood industry was worth approximately 18.5 billion dollars.[32] In his text *Blood: An Epic History of Medicine and Commerce,* Douglas Starr made a striking comparison between blood and oil, observing that a "barrel of crude oil . . . sells for about $13 at this writing. The same quantity of whole blood, in its 'crude' state, would sell for more than $20,000."[33] At the time, an individual unit of blood was worth about $150 to $200. Testing each unit for diseases cost between $25 and $35, not including expenses for training employees and basic quality control.[34] Blood is a serious business, and a costly one at that.

Ironically, while blood products constitute a multi-billion-dollar industry, today contributors of blood are almost universally volunteers.[35] The second event that had a tremendous impact on the blood industry was the emphasis on courting unpaid donors. For many years, there were competing systems of attracting donors. Some benevolent organizations attracted volunteers by appealing to nationalism, altruism, and the bonds of community. For decades, however, there were also blood-for-profit centers, which came to fruition in the mid-1950s. These centers paid donors a small fee for their services and had a tense relationship with some medical communities because of their poor collection procedures and unsanitary blood samples.[36] All that began to change in 1970 when Richard Titmuss published his influential text on the blood-donor system, *The Gift Relationship.* Here he argued that cultural understandings of blood and its worth influenced the safety of the blood supply. People who thought of blood as a gift and not a commodity were less likely to infect the blood supply, because they were giving altruistically, not because they wanted money for drugs or alcohol. According to Titmuss, buying blood was deleterious because it attracted populations that were more likely to abuse substances and carry sexually transmitted diseases. At the time Titmuss argued that these variables were especially significant since, according to his disputed study, only 10 percent of donated blood came from volunteers.[37]

Although Titmuss's project has received scrutiny for its unreliable data and poor understanding of people's desire for cultural inclusion, his study caught the attention of government officials, prompting the implementation of numerous health measures. The federal government imposed regulations that included a mandatory label distinction between commercial and donated blood. Volunteer systems grew to be the preferred method of donation, and populations that were paid for their fluids were seen as more likely to abuse drugs and to have a higher incidence of disease.[38] As a direct result, the system converted to being almost entirely voluntary, as hospitals and members of the blood services industry attempted to avoid lawsuits stemming from purchased blood. Volunteers were a necessity, rhetorically constructed as civic minded, free of disease, and irreplaceable.

As blood science became more technologically savvy and safety measures increasingly stringent, the nation was hit by one of the most deadly epidemics in recorded history. The onset of AIDS and the government's failure to respond shook the altruistic donation system at its foundation. Almost overnight the metaphor for engaged national identity morphed into a material and symbolic global nightmare.

THE RHETORICAL DIVIDE:
"PUBLIC HEALTH" VERSUS "CIVIL RIGHTS"

Removed several decades from the panic that initially characterized AIDS, it is easier today to make the case that the blood-donor ban should be abolished. Scientific methods for screening out dangerous contagions in blood have proven overwhelmingly effective and every major authority on blood donation agrees that the supply is safer today than at any other point in its history. The ARC assures the public that the chance of contracting HIV from donated blood is 1 in 1.5 million. They claim to make "every effort to recruit a healthy population of volunteer blood donors." The agency discards about 2 percent of the fluids it collects annually because of test results, although "only a fraction of those pose a threat and a true health risk."[39]

In the early 1980s proclamations about risk were not so transparent. In fact, by all accounts safeguards to the blood supply were imposed months later than they should have been. The scientific community faced a convoluted situation that demanded immediate judgment, with little medical evidence or government support. Along with the stigmatizing of gay men, health officials had to consider the safety of the nation's entire blood supply, including the lives of transfusion recipients and hemophiliacs. They faced competing social and economic responsibilities that typically accompany the implementation of controversial policies and widespread health regulations. Decision makers were confronted with a number of disparate variables, some of which supported the ban, others of which did not. As one writer explained: "Because fewer than ten out of more than eight-hundred cases of AIDS were linked to blood transfusions at the time, because more than ten million units of blood were transfused annually, and because concerns were expressed whether questions regarding a donor's sexual preference might be considered an invasion of privacy, there was no consensus in the medical community as to how to proceed."[40] The reluctance to impose safety measures was one of the many bureaucratic disasters in the early stages of containment. The lack of action on the part of the government prior to policy implementation had catastrophic effects, resulting in a reported 4,833 cases of HIV infection through blood transfusions.[41]

Along with the circumstances mentioned above, in several parts of the country gay donors were considered a vital population for collecting blood, and several organizations were reluctant to implement exclusionary measures. In San Francisco, gay blood donors were valued because they were generally "well educated and civic-minded," providing about a fifth of the supply to some blood banks.[42] At a time of declining donor rates, gay men remained a consistent and loyal source of blood products in several parts of the country. Although the generalization of being "well educated" echoes the stereotype that gay men are upper-middle class and have disproportionate amounts of disposable income, it nevertheless calls attention to the importance of gay donors in many communities.

Following extended deliberation the FDA took the initial steps of imposing the ban in March 1983. A number of male hemophiliacs and an infant were diagnosed with HIV, and the blood products used were traced to gay men.[43] The agencies were faced with the unthinkable—that HIV was traveling through the national blood supply. It threatened to infect the nation's hemophiliac population, many of whom were dependent on blood products to produce Factor VIII, a clotting agent that allowed them to live free from the bodily pain induced by hemophilia. An unidentified amount of tainted blood also stood to wreak havoc in the nation's hospitals, where thousands of operations and standard blood transfusions took place on a daily basis.

The PHS recommended all blood collection centers institute a question in their donor screening forms to phase out members of so-called high-risk groups. While the original government intervention did not specify what screening procedures to incorporate to ascertain sexual behavior, it did demand immediate intervention. The orders quickly morphed in the question that asks: "are you a male that has had sexual contact with another male, even once, since 1977?" Any person who answered affirmatively would be permanently banned from contributing blood. Adding the question to the forms was seen as the most effective and inexpensive method of securing the blood supply. While health officials were partially concerned the ban would ignite tempers in the gay community, "public safety" threatened by the increased numbers of HIV exposure took precedent over claims to privacy and inclusion. James Curran, the head of AIDS research at the Center for Disease Control (CDC), bluntly stated, "the medical problem is more important than the civil rights issue."[44] This controversial sentiment continues to circulate today, even by some queer men.[45]

The tension that was produced between "civil rights" and "public health" has become a prominent theme of the discourse both in the medical community and among LGBT rights advocates. In an ARC memo dated February 5, 1983, one official wrote, "Legally, it would seem that we are open to suit in any event i.e. [*sic*] by the gays if we attempt to exclude them, by patients who might contacts [*sic*] AIDS if we don't make every attempt to exclude gays."[46] In the end, broad exclusions were permitted because epidemiological evidence could support controversial decision making.[47] Commenting on this tension, one legal analyst explained: "To public health policy makers in the United States, the risk of harm associated with HIV, of acquiring a fatal or potentially fatal disease from a blood transfusion, far outweighs the costs of pre- and post-donation screening or any consequent infringement on liberty interests or personal autonomy in denying someone the opportunity to donate blood."[48] The word "opportunity" is a key term here. There are no constitutional provisions that afford one the right to donate blood. While the ARC and other blood agencies continually push for volunteers, they are under no obligation to accept donations from all who are willing to give.[49] When Dr. Curran referenced the "civil rights issue," it was partially accurate, but a moot point in many regards. Nonetheless, the debate has come to be historically framed in public memory as a struggle between "public health" and "civil rights." One text on HIV and the blood supply captures this theme succinctly, stating that the "gay community saw donor questioning as an infringement of their rights. The CDC viewed it as the sole means of protecting the public health at the time."[50]

The blood ban forced competing perspectives on the ethics of altruism and the relationship between individuals and the communities they inhabit. While there is no inherent right to donate blood, there was much concern over excluding a large segment of the population. This attention to prohibitions signals a cultural acknowledgment of the direct connection that is present between the ritual of blood donation and the constitutive nature of civic engagement. As a result, the medical community had to rhetorically establish that queer men could best practice citizenship by withholding donations. This was accomplished in large part through the rhetorical schism constructed between "public health" and "civil rights."

The phrase "public health" is especially potent, as it combines the rhetorical force of an idealized communal sphere (public) with a powerful God-term (health). While there are multiple ways of defining the term "public," it is most generally used in healthcare matters to mean something of "concern for

all people," though this broad positioning invites oversight and marginalization.[51] Like many epidemics, in the early days of AIDS the act of blood donation could be conceived of as a "public" health crisis only to the extent that
meanings were conceptualized largely outside the realm of "public" knowledge. This gave rise to what Paula Triechler has termed an "epidemic of sig-
nification," in which a narrow understanding of the AIDS crisis developed,
often under the guise of scientific information, simultaneously stigmatizing
queer men and neglecting the problems confronting them. Indeed, a "public"
crisis gained capital only when it was determined that heterosexuals would be
at risk for contracting AIDS. Triechler notes, after reports that heterosexuals
were susceptible to AIDS, "what had changed was not 'the facts' but the way
in which they were now used to construct the AIDS text and the meanings
that we were now allowed—indeed, at least encouraged—to read from that
text."[52] The public fight against AIDS slowly became articulated with the impulses of liberal democracy and an effort was made to say "we're all equally
at risk" and "we're all in this together."[53] For queer men, that public sacrifice
included, and continues to involve, the self-exclusion of being a blood donor
in their communities.

The degree to which the "public" has been conceived of as an idealized
sphere that tends to exclude those on the fringes of society has gained significant attention from scholars.[54] AIDS activists had to fight hard for public
acknowledgment of the epidemic and those most victimized by its wrath.[55]
Indeed, President Reagan didn't even acknowledge the epidemic publicly
until 1987, long after it had been determined that this syndrome would alter
the global landscape. Cindy Patton reminds readers that "the way the story
of AIDS is told has . . . great effect on the acceptability of policies that are
promoted within that story's narrative reach."[56] The deaths of thousands of
gay men went unnoticed by the government for years because they were
"not recognized as constituents of the (now infamously phrased) 'general
population.'"[57]

The term "public" is reinforced by the rhetorical force of the term "health."
This single word flexes tremendous discursive muscle as it constitutes perhaps
one of the most powerful God-terms in Western cultures. "Health" functions to reinforce mythic notions of the pure nation-state and the "biological
responsibilities" that accompany citizenship in that space.[58] Troy Duster observes that public health "discourse is always in terms of the medical, health,
and scientific benefits, skewing the grounds upon which an informed debate
about other social, cultural, and political questions can arise."[59] In some ways,
the phrase "public health" takes on the qualities of an ideograph in the medical
community, as such an expression represents "in condensed form the norma-

tive, collective commitments of the members of a public" typically appearing in arguments as "the necessary motivations or justifications for action performed in the name of the public."[60]

While "public health" is a dominant frame in the debate surrounding the blood ban, the phrase "civil rights" also carries substantial cultural capital. However, despite the potentially productive appropriation of "civil rights," the individual focus that is associated with equality free of discrimination is counterproductive in a discourse that stresses relationships in a blood ritual. There should be no mistaking the fact that giving blood is above and beyond all else a privilege, not a protected right. "Civil rights" implies that which is inalienable and necessary for sustaining a healthy democratic culture by protecting specific personal freedoms. Blood donation, while a source of pride and national identification, is difficult to claim as essential to an individual's well-being. It is unlike job security and equal housing opportunities in that it does not affect the quotidian life of the minority represented in the social equation. In fact, the invocation of "civil rights" is, in many ways, politically disempowering. It implies political access and legal recognition, not "cultural acceptance, social transformation, understanding, and liberation."[61]

The term "civil rights" has always had a tenuous relationship with the gay community. The political right-wing has long purported that gays and lesbians are already afforded "civil rights" and have no "immutable" characteristics that would enable them the protections offered to other marginalized citizens. The appeal to a rights-based discourse is easy enough to understand. Patricia Ewick and Susan Silbey point out that in claiming a legal "right": "a person crystallizes experience in a set of abstractions that invoke connection and deference that have been empirically unavailable, hence the need to invoke the legal claim of right. Nonetheless, the label 'right' authorizes and legitimates the imagining of association and community that is denied in practice."[62] Rather than acknowledge denied access to some civic rituals and economic incongruities, our political system has long assumed that gays and lesbians could hide their sexualities and garner the rights they need invisibly. This can be complicated for a number of reasons, including, for example, the implementation of policies (such as a blood-donor screening) that directly inquire about a person's sexual practices.

Of course, it is tempting for gay rights activists to embrace the rhetoric of secular argument that has provided a catalyst for numerous LGBT causes. James Darsey is wise to remind us, however, that such rhetoric "is almost apolitical . . . in that it addresses the multitude as a mass of individuals, not as a political unity. Its appeal is not to *de cive* but to each person as the maker of his or her own destiny."[63] In the ritual of blood donation such individuality is discounted because personal gain is viewed as secondary to the fate awaiting the person receiving the gift of life. Recipients are placed in a position of vulnerability, relying on an intermediary system that can be trusted to determine who is best qualified to save lives. Herein lays the centerpiece of the debate—delimiting who is allowed to act with *maximum consciousness* as a member of the civic culture.

This muddy tension between "rights" and "privileges" is illustrated clearly in the appeals of the Gay and Lesbian Medical Association, one of the few LGBT organizations who have consistently advocated for the modification of deferral policies. They argue that the "guidelines are commonly defended with the statement that giving blood is a privilege, not a right, a statement that flies in the face of the fact that giving blood has always been promoted as a responsibility of all citizens of the U.S."[64] As true as these claims may be, "privilege" and "responsibility" are literally separated by the concept of "rights" in this statement, resituating their argument within a frame that will ultimately work against them. The group's assertions would benefit from a distancing of terminology that incorporates a rights-based vocabulary as such language does little more than reinforce the classification schema their adversaries are promoting.

Although historical accounts often construe the gay rights movement as largely unified around the issue of civil rights, the blood ban actually divided many leaders in the gay community.[65] While some immediately began to suggest self-deferrals, others maintained that overgeneralizing gay male sexual behavior was a dangerous practice. As documented by Randy Shilts, some groups such as the Bay Area Physicians for Human Rights and the American Association of Physicians for Human Rights were encouraging gay men to exclude themselves from the donation process. In return, some blood banks withheld from soliciting a donor's sexual orientation, asking instead if people had symptoms such as swollen lymph nodes and night sweats.[66] Conversely, groups such as the National Gay Task Force opposed screening questionnaires on the grounds that they invaded privacy and reinforced negative stereotypes of gay men. At the end of the day, most groups accepted the donor exclusion policies, thinking that new blood technologies and HIV tests would eventually render invasive questions about sexuality unnecessary.

Compounding the tension between public health and personal liberties were cultural narratives that pitted gay identity against "victimized populations." While inclusion in the ritual of giving blood was seen as an important producer of cultural identity, this "right" was situated against the threat of contaminating the bodies of other people. Prior to the implementation of the deferral policies, spokespeople from the National Hemophilia Foundation began expressing concerns that groups such as the National Gay Task Force were being unreasonable in their push to keep gay men a consistent part of the donor pool. One representative commented, "They may want to protect their rights, but what about the hemophiliacs' right to life?"[67] The tension between LGBT groups and the hemophiliac lobby continues today and is often used to justify policies by decision makers. The false dilemma of the state having to choose one side over the other rather than pursue alternative policy options is compounded by a discourse of equality that pits two groups against each other, a frequent pattern in American political history.

Three years into Reagan's first term stories about gay men who continued to donate blood despite the ban began to circulate as national panic ensued. In Austin, Texas, a gay man named Christopher Whitfield died in the fall of 1983, becoming the city's first recognized AIDS victim. Recalling the name, one health worker looked up Whitfield's medical background only to discover that he had donated plasma forty-eight times. According to these officials Whitfield had no visible symptoms of AIDS when donating and had lied to officials about being a member of a "high-risk group."[68] Various research reports indicated gay men lied about their sexual orientation and their sexual history, or made incorrect assumptions about the accuracy of testing procedures used to screen blood.[69] Some health officials even worried that gay men would donate out of spite, engaging in a type of "blood terrorism."[70]

Examples of gay men who donated "contaminated" blood, knowingly or not, stood in sharp contrast to the narrative told of people who received it for transfusions. These were innocent victims who had fallen prey to the "fast and loose lifestyles" of unhealthy donors. Stories about mothers, babies, teenagers, and hemophiliacs who were contracting HIV from blood products began circulating in the media. In California, the Blood Safety Act was named after Paul Gann, a man who died from HIV/AIDS complications after he was given a transfusion.[71] So extensive was the blood scare that in 1987 a poll conducted by the American Association of Blood Banks (AABB) found that 27 percent of the people they surveyed thought they could get AIDS from *donating* blood.[72] The ritual of blood donation no longer constituted a positive enactment of citizenship—it instead represented death.

As the AIDS crisis grew to pandemic proportions, the issue of donor exclusion policies quickly disappeared into the background of public discussion. While it continued to gain sporadic attention from public health academics and medical officials in government agencies, the issue of banned blood was quickly replaced by other pressing needs. With containment methods well underway, prevention measures geared toward heterosexual communities, such as sex education, took the national spotlight. When the FDA revisited the donor deferral measures ten years following the initial moratorium, it was framed as being "simply too hot to handle" and received almost no attention from the popular press.[73]

In addition, the subject matter of blood donation all but disappeared from the rhetoric of the gay rights movement as advocates turned their attention to issues such as gays in the military, civil unions (and later same-sex marriage), mediated representations, and AIDS education. Who could blame movement organizers for being hesitant? After all, gays were placed in the precarious position of being blamed for the unfolding epidemic. Their identities became articulated with the dangers of AIDS in a number of popular cultural forms including television, film, and in the halls of Congress. In the midst of a cultural panic where people were quick to assign responsibility for the syndrome, who would want to offer more fuel for the fire of antigay forces? Of course, gay and lesbian groups were also largely left to their own devices for raising awareness among queer populations about AIDS. Few resources were available for pushing such a controversial issue at such a difficult time.[74]

REVISITING THE RHETORIC OF THE BLOOD BAN

In the years 1997 and 2000, the issue of blood-donor deferrals for men who have sex with other men was raised, and by a close vote the BPAC upheld the ban.[75] Despite the assurances of the CDC, the FDA, and the ARC that testing measures screen out all contagions, the BPAC voted against revoking exclusionary policies. Despite all the safe-sex education measures implemented throughout the country, no changes were made. Despite blood protection acts and federal policies that protect blood banks and donation centers from lawsuits, the BPAC upheld the mandatory ban.[76] Despite the fact that it is now well known that heterosexuals can also contract, carry, and spread HIV (and that they have unsafe, promiscuous, and random sex), the panel sustained this discriminatory policy by using science as a convenient rhetorical vehicle for their decision.

Years later, in the spring of 2006 the ARC at long last joined America's Blood Centers and the American Association of Blood Banks (collectively being the three agencies that collect almost all donated blood in the United States) in calling for an end to the indefinite deferral measure. Significantly, however, officials at the ARC were content on allowing the FDA to maintain incongruous standards between male donors who acknowledged same-sex sexual activity and those who did not. Despite the seeming progress in their newly adopted position, the ARC endorsed a policy change that would continue to defer men who have sex with other men if they reported engaging in *any* sexual behavior within the last year. The policy again overlooked men who practiced safe sex or were involved in monogamous relationships, maintaining discrepancies between queer donors and heterosexuals. Men who have sex with other men in *any* capacity are still equivocal to the most unsafe of sexual practices. In May 2007 the FDA reiterated its support for the ban. Without offering any reason for this sudden announcement, a permanent, lifetime ban remains in place for queer men. Less than a year later the head of the FDA again defended the ban to a congressional subcommittee.

Scientific "truths" employed by the government to produce a hierarchy of healthy, and thus valued, citizens must be questioned. Although the blood ban has been elided in public conversations, it is time to reincorporate it more forcefully into discourses emphasizing queer citizenship. Sexuality in this debate has too long been defined by institutions that posit knowledge about queer bodies that does little more than eviscerate the trust, goodwill, and sacrifices made by citizens.[77] Eve Sedgwick has argued that "homosexuality," the term consistently employed in official rhetorics, has continually been represented as self-evident in the discourses that define it.[78] Despite the many strides made by LGBT people, these supposedly self-evident truths continue to plague civic identities, even when logical contradictions about the nature of queer citizens materialize. However, these inconsistencies in official conceptions of sexuality do not call into question the cultural legitimacy of false claims made about gays and lesbians. In fact, contradictions often operate simultaneously to reinforce power structures. For example, discourses that frame the blood ban closely parallel Sedgwick's formulation that gay men are positioned both as the border-crossers of gender and as radical separatists. These incongruities do not render the discourse powerless, but serve to ensure incoherent understandings of gay men.[79] The elasticity of sexuality and gender imaginaries ensure that queer men can be recognized as a threat and insignificant at the same time.

In her text *The Queen of America Goes to Washington City,* Lauren Berlant argues that AIDS has figured prominently in shaping conceptions of citizenship in the United States. The manner in which citizenship is projected no longer envisions people as having lives in progress, but imagines "sexuality in the shadow of deaths to be avoided."[80] Berlant explains, "AIDS has made it possible to draw an absolute public boundary between U.S. citizens and gay people."[81] This unnatural schism positions an entire class of people to live as strangers in their own communities, treated not with hospitality and respect, but hostility and retaliation. This rift has a chilling effect on identity groups such as gay and lesbians, who are often asked to withhold or censor their anger because they are not viewed, in Berlant's words, "as productive."[82] Rather than depict collective grievances as based on principles and sound reasoning, the LGBT community is often positioned by ruling parties and the media as basing their views on mere passions, posing a threat to the stability of a rational democratic culture.

At one point in time, the blood ban against men who have sex with men was arguably reasonable. Even as we should remain suspicious of such drastic institutional measures, the fact remains that there was little knowledge about AIDS, people were dying, and the government's initial response was abhorrent. However, we now know volumes about HIV and its modes of transmission and have reliable testing methods for blood.[83] The once moral dilemma we faced has been replaced by the promises of safe-sex education and the work of blood science. Today, innumerable gay, bisexual, and queer men are marginalized at all costs. The ARC continually asserts the need for more volunteers, as the national blood supply seems to be in a perpetual state of crisis. Despite these pleas, scores of men are prevented from participating in one of the most altruistic and necessary forms of civic engagement. This cultural script needs to be revised, and the blood ban is a productive point at which to start rewriting notions of citizenship and the relationships we should have with one another.

The solution, however, is not as simple as one might at first think. Activists who oppose the blood ban face novel forms of cultural and ideological exclusion. What is cause for concern is not simply that queer men are being stigmatized through the exclusion of their blood. Rather, it is the complex cultural disciplining of their bodies that becomes most disturbing when faced with this disconcerting blood-ban rhetoric. The cultural recourse for queer men to be included in communities remains elusive while institutions continue to conspire against these citizens in frightening ways. Gay rights advocates, for example, have faced numerous institutional obstacles when challenging the ARC, which collects approximately half of all blood in the United States.[84] Although blood drives are typically local events, and donation centers are usually located in visible segments of a community, the ARC is not a local agency. As a "patriot society," it acts as a federally chartered corporation for the United States government. While it remains a separate and distinct institution from the state, subject to lawsuits from private citizens, the organization is afforded important protections.[85] Despite the fact the ARC is not granted sovereign immunity, it is granted federal jurisdiction in all lawsuits.[86] The Supreme Court has concluded that the ARC's Charter "provides original federal jurisdiction for all cases in which the Red Cross is a party."[87] This is alarming because claims to state and local laws "have the capacity to be tried in federal court, regardless of diversity" or questions of jurisdiction.[88]

In other words, local ordinances and state laws can be rendered powerless because policies are subject to review by blanket federal standards that may disregard variations in regulation and principle.

Federal courts typically exhibit tremendous deference to federal guidelines and regulations, making it difficult for blood-ban opponents to litigate their causes.[89] There is little recourse for those who operate on the local level, as federal courts are insulated from popular election and from juries that could be sympathetic to residents with whom they may be acquainted. It presents a striking question for critics: how should people approach a legal system constructed to shield institutions that inhibit a person's desire to be included fully in the fabric of the cultural identity of citizenship on a federal level? This dilemma is especially troubling for activists fighting against the mentality that guides the blood ban. There are no federal protections for gays and lesbians, no constitutional or legislative measures that shelter them from various forms of discrimination, whether they pertain to "civil rights" or cultural inscriptions of citizenship. Individuals who are being discriminated against necessarily turn to local ordinances that might offer some form of comfort and support in the face of adversity. But here we are faced with a precarious situation. Even if a citizen wanted to call into question the degree to which a local ARC action violates the terms of local protection policies, the organization is federally insulated from legal actions, regardless of the merit of the claims being made. It would require redress on a federal level, which disregards the local values goading the plaintiff, discounts the queer identities of the men wishing to donate blood, and relegates discussions back to issues of "civil rights," which would prove unproductive for activists.

Clearly, these issues present a pressing need to explore the rigid contours of the blood ban and search for viable alternatives to the erroneously destructive policies. This study seeks to reinvigorate the debate surrounding the blood ban by probing the complex rhetorical features of the exclusionary measures. *Banning Queer Blood* speaks to issues of citizenship and democratic practice, questioning the perpetual myths that plague the gay community, passed down by injurious discourses and unsound epidemiological data. National policies can have a stark impact on the quotidian production of citizenship, especially in the ritual space of blood donation. The subordination of queer identity in these discourses exists not in the abstract, but with material consequences in local communities. In recent years queer students at a university where I conducted interviews for this book, for example, have been asked to run aspects of blood drives, such as volunteering to hand out cookies, in place of acting as donors. Their marginalization, centrally featured at the ritual site, exemplifies the contempt collection agencies have for their civic capabilities and sacrifices.

QUEERING THE RHETORIC OF THE BLOOD BAN

The themes outlined in this chapter, which resurface throughout the text, are informed by many voices in the humanities. *Banning Queer Blood* draws from conversations taking place in cultural studies, rhetorical theory, queer theory, and gay and lesbian studies. This diverse, interdisciplinary archive enhances understandings of discourses that stigmatize and situate queer bodies as a threat to the polity. With their emphases on the everyday, norms, language, agency, and subjects, the fields of rhetorical studies and cultural studies have left clear footprints on this project. Like the tenants of queer theory, rhetorical and cultural studies have long sustained a healthy distrust of Platonic conceptions of truth. Since the days of the Sophists in ancient Greece, the idea that truth is a radically contingent process, not a monolithic state of being, has been a hallmark of rhetorical studies. Throughout this text, there is a consistent engagement with the rhetorical constitution of identities and how those identities come into being via tropes, metaphors, narratives, rituals, and myths. Indeed, rhetorical studies share many commonplaces with queer theory: each is obsessed with lived culture; each highlights the performative nature of identity and the body; each is grounded in the language of political culture and its manifestations; and each is concerned with the deployment of citizenship.

This study also rests at the fulcrum of LGBT studies and queer theory. LGBT studies' embrace of visibility politics and push for structural inclusion and civil rights is often placed in opposition to the major tenants of queer theory, which assumes the evasion of an essential identity. Advocates of queer theory warn of the dangers associated with normalization, the pitfalls of institutional assimilation, and the hazards inherent in liberation politics. This analysis borrows heavily from both camps, recognizing that LGBT studies and queer theory have as much to offer each other as they do to this project. As Michael Warner explains, these "rhetorics belong not to different epochs, or to different populations, but to different contexts."[90] Queer theory, in other words, cannot point to the detriment of normalization without a sustained movement that produces a significant set of discourses. In this way, queer theory is dependent on long-standing and emerging rhetorics developed in traditional movements. Conversely, with increased appeals to national inclusion, queer theory offers LGBT studies an effective check on movement political strategies. Far from being a reactive form of scholarship, queer theory can offer insightful alternatives to diabolically heterosexist politics, attempting to alter the frames through which people understand issues and events. In this manner gay and lesbian scholarship, as well as queer theory, are productive in as much as they seek to forge new spaces for understanding civic identity and its discontents.

In the rhetoric of the blood ban, for example, it is important to probe how the FDA has traditionally envisioned sexual identity in order to question the claims that it is advancing. Scientists and bureaucrats who have a heavy hand in the development of deferral policies are careful not to employ terms such as "gay" when conversing about the stigmatizing regulations. Instead, they employ the more sanitized term, "men who have sex with other men," clinically cleansing the identities that "gay" implies. Such a phrase is "queer" in that it does not assume a stable identity, but also runs the risk of conflating notions of identity into singular instances of behavior. The deployment of MSM (men who have sex with other men) as a phrase is perhaps most disheartening because of its seeming utopian potential. LGBT advocates have long searched for inclusive terms that might more fully encapsulate the range of experiences available to us. While MSM does not adequately account for desire, it might otherwise be a useful heuristic for imagining queer lives. Unfortunately the positioning of MSM by the state is not utilized in a manner that would enable queers to become more active and lively civic participants.

There is little doubt that queer men have been isolated from their communities by their exclusion from donating blood. On this note, I am confident in my belief that queer men should be allowed to donate to the national supply. At the same time, following the maxims of queer theory, I recognize that lifting the ban, "normalizing" the blood of the queer citizen, will not offer a purified "liberation" to the populations that the blood ban is most violently geared toward. Again, queer theorists continually caution against the limitations of "normalization" fabricated by the state and its numerous agencies. Such discourses produce "truths" that perpetually marginalize and victimize people who fail to uphold cultural norms.

Some critics have suggested that the concepts of "citizenship" and "queer" are themselves antithetical, with citizenship always acting upon normalizing discourses that legitimize state interests. Amy Brandzel, for example, argues that "queers, especially those who are privileged and well off enough to do so, should refuse citizenship."[91] Although Brandzel's goal of subverting normativity is laudable, such analyses rarely engage the more important question of how one might reject *being* a citizen in all of its multifarious forms. Those who are "privileged" in American culture, in particular, have capitalized on their positions as citizen actors; implying they can live as privileged, but not citizens, seems to accomplish little for those who cannot enact their citizenship to start. Attempts to reject that identity should be viewed with skepticism, not mere admiration. Often, such critiques overlook the intersectional nature of "queer," homogenizing the relationships that could be articulated between identity, citizenship, and resistance. Nonetheless, these writers also offer an important cautionary flag for those overly eager to entertain invitations for cultural assimilation.

Queer critics recognize the recalcitrance that is placed on identities when they are situated in public deliberations that typically marginalize them. Limits are set on that which is considered normal and acceptable to the imagined general public, with some bodies being included and others excluded. Scholars who adopt a queer perspective strive to push for a more robust and agonistic discussion by highlighting the limits of such normalization. While queer men may one day be allowed to donate blood, queer critics would warn that the prohibitions directed toward those who engage in "unsafe behaviors" may continue to carry more stigma than the "unsafe" acts of heterosexuals. What degree of bodily monitoring must transpire before queer men have convinced government officials that they are worthy of being citizens? What do gay men give up in order to be a part of a polity that allowed so many of them to die? This is not to suggest that these issues are clear cut, have proscribed answers, or can be easily understood—quite the opposite is true. However, the convoluted nature of these questions, coupled with the dangers of subscribing to an ideology that situates queer citizenship as lethal, necessitates a perspective that challenges the ontological positioning of such identities in this treacherous discourse.

This is also not to say that queer theory must provide all the answers. Queer theory, like any discipline, cannot purport to know what it will discover prior to approaching the complex and contingent discourses it is engaging. In many ways the blood ban advances our understandings of queer theory and community as it demarcates what is, and is not, tolerable to our contemporary political cultures. As Berlant and Warner explain, AIDS taught gay people not to "assume a social environment of community and of support for legitimate politics. Far from preexisting as sources of activism and critical commentary, communities of support had to be created by a public labor."[92] Queer theory brings together those realms which appear distinct and articulates their ability to conceive that which is normal in performances of citizenship. From a heuristic standpoint, these perspectives will help delimit complex cultural forms and offer productive strategies for recuperating the civic identities of queer men.

PLAN OF THE VOLUME

Dissecting the discursive corpus of the blood ban requires focus on an array of divergent and overlapping rhetorics. As such, *Banning Queer Blood* concentrates on a number of social norms and performative acts of citizenship that are concurrently tied to and separated from queer identity. Exploring the intricate features of the blood ban necessitates an investigation not only of stigmatization, but also the relationship between blood, sexuality, and political culture, the apparatus of memory that situates the ban, the rhetorical construction of bodies in scientific epistemologies, and the resistance set forth by queer communities.

Accordingly, chapter 2 engages the symbolic significance of blood and its relationship to sexuality and national identity. Building off of a legal case in which a gay blood donor was charged with "negligent misrepresentation," I argue that the image of the queer man in relation to blood and nationhood is always already condemned to such positioning. Using Foucault's discussion of bio-politics to examine the rhetorical strategies of state discourses, I probe the fabrication of an idealized citizen that is placed in contrast to the imagined queer body. The intertwining tropes of the "reproductive citizen" and the "sacrificial citizen" proffer insight into government visions of queer men in the political order. The queer citizen is a carefully articulated abjection, having a strong internal presence in the social body, but also read as a foreign entity in polity. The threat posed by the shadow of the queer man is exemplified in the donor deferral question, which is closely scrutinized at the chapter's conclusion.

The discursive mechanisms that maintain the blood ban are rooted in contemporary recollections of the initial AIDS crisis. As such, gauging how the ban has been remembered in contemporary cultural rhetorics is the focus of the third chapter. Two primary media texts, *And the Band Played On* and *Red Gold: The Epic Story of Blood,* are incorporated to inspect how citizens are encouraged to recall the blood supply disasters of the early 1980s. Competing notions of queer sexuality permeate this memory, strongly mediated by gendered figures. The first is the matriarch, infected by a blood donor who was unaware of his HIV status. The second is the image of the hemophiliac, always positioned as a docile body against the proud, masculine gay mob that actively ignores the dangers of AIDS. This articulation of "unaware" and "acting in maximum consciousness" upholds contemporary rhetorics situating queer men as living in social denial, of knowing, but refusing to acknowledge, their propensity for contracting and transmitting HIV/AIDS.

The power of science and public health to prolong the ban occupies the heart of chapter 4. At the center of this chapter are three government transcripts detailing deliberative forums where possible changes to the ban were contemplated. Two of the texts stem from BPAC meetings held in December 1997 and September 2000. The third is an account of an FDA meeting called to discuss potential alterations to the ban in light of new research indicating progress in the fight against HIV. Although the transcripts signal that technological progress has secured the blood supply, sexuality is rendered more potent than scientific advancements. Consistently, these deliberations depict queer men as contagions, more prone to new and dangerous maladies, as exemplified by the committee's troubling metaphors, evidence, and supposed methodological process.

While health officials and scientists represent these citizens as hazardous, queer donors understand themselves as altruistic volunteers who are conscientious about their health and the well-being of others. Chapter 5 employs interviewing research to explore the ways queer men view their place in the ritual of giving blood. Men who both "passed" to contribute blood, as well as those who protested when turned away, were interviewed. Together, these two groups of men demonstrate a dialogical mode of resistance that offers support for expunging the deferral measure. When read collectively, these interviews show that contaminated queer blood is not slipping into the system.

Drawing on the analytical details of the pages that precede it, the concluding chapter calls for a reconstitution of the blood-ban debate, asserting a reconfiguration of the framework traditionally utilized to understand queer citizens and blood donation. Advocating the themes of "refusal," "curiosity," and "innovation," several propositions are advanced: that the questionnaires must be reformulated, that queer lobbies must further protest the ban, and that everyday resistance must persist. The inclusion of queer men would reinvigorate the polis in productive ways by strengthening social bonds, generating volunteers, and saving lives.

Banning Queer Blood scrutinizes how the blood ban is rhetorically manifest in seemingly diffuse discourses. Ultimately this study argues that such policies inhibit our ability to act with maximum consciousness by reproducing outdated and injurious conceptions of queer citizens. However, it also aspires for a transformative cultural politics that refuses unwarranted disciplinary actions. The harm engendered by the ban can be undone, but only with commitment to a cultural politics that values difference. There is little doubt that presumption currently rests with heterosexism and the state. But the burden of proof is increasingly weighing on the shoulders of a few health officials who cannot sustain these blatantly discriminatory practices. The possibilities for reimagining citizenship in the ritual site of blood sacrifice have already begun to take shape. This book furthers the conversation with the hope that all people will be treated fairly, fortifying the health and goodwill of citizens and the democracy we inhabit.

2
Articulating Abjection
Negating Citizenships of Sacrifice and Reproduction

In the summer of 2002, officials at the Canadian Blood Services (CBS) were taunted by an anonymous gay man who claimed to be donating to the national supply.[1] Frustrated with policies that prohibited him from contributing blood, the unknown citizen sent scornful notes to agency administrators: "I am a gay man and have been involved in a long-term, committed relationship. . . . Both my partner and myself have been tested for the HIV virus and are both negative, and intend to stay that way. We are both honest people, and are both blood donors."[2] Although bitter, the man's words were scarcely radical. He appealed to being clean, monogamous, and health conscious, not infected, promiscuous, and potentially dangerous. Nonetheless, the heckling disturbed the powers-that-be at the regulatory state agency. Canada employs the same deferral question for men who have sex with other men as the United States and similarly maintains an identical lifetime ban. If this man and his partner were in fact donating the "juice of life," they were violating health regulations implemented to keep the blood supply free of "high-risk" populations. An investigation ensued and eventually organization officials located the couple after a supreme court justice ordered an internet service provider to release the IP address attached to the antagonistic e-mail messages.

The CBS filed suit against the man known only as "John Doe," citing negligent misrepresentation and seeking $175,000 in damages. The agency claimed this money would be used to track down citizens who may have received the men's blood and to offer them free HIV tests. Citing the seriousness of the offense, one official for the CBS explained to the press that "the recipients of blood products made from his donations had a right to the safest, highest blood-quality products we can provide."[3]

The disconnect in logic between "John Doe" and CBS is fairly easy to discern. There is no consideration by CBS that this man might be healthy. There is no confirmation that he had been in a long-term relationship. There is no attempt to quell public fears by offering the two men HIV tests and not countless others who think they may have received their blood, possibly panicking because of the mythologies that circulate about gay male sexuality.[4] The court order clearly illustrated, in the words of CBS, that "public health trumps privacy concerns," even if public health never surfaces as an issue.[5] But what we can learn most from this incident lies not simply in the incommensurability of warring factions, but in a follow-up story just one month later. As it turns out, Mr. Doe inspired a copycat.

Just weeks after "John Doe" made his court appearance, a second man, called "John Doe II" by Canadian officials, started sending electronic messages to the government alleging to be disease free, but violating policies by giving blood. In his correspondence, he encouraged thousands of banned blood donors to come forward and demand an end to the double standard. "Why don't you automatically assume that all straight people have syphilis, gonorrhea, and hepatitis?" he asked, adding, "Because your policy is based in ignorance, hate and stupidity. It was you fuckwits who spread AIDS and hepatitis in the 1980s by not testing the blood supply. It was not the donors."[6]

Although the government initially pursued the second rabble-rouser, they quickly dismissed his case. Noting that his e-mail was coming from an untraceable source outside national borders, officials rejected the idea that "John Doe II" was a genuine menace, even if his words were considerably more adverse than his predecessor. But the degree to which one of these men was so severely disciplined and the other so swiftly disregarded is telling. It signals a tacit affiliation of nation, blood, and notions of civic identity. The positioning of the second man as clearly outside the body politic with little regard for his proximity to its boundaries or the degree to which his rhetoric might gain traction is revealing in that it illustrates a relationship that has more to do with epistemological insecurity and disciplinary regimen than claims to sanctuary and sound mind. They didn't prosecute "John Doe" because he was dangerous—they did it because he violated the discursive purity of civic embodiment necessary for the production of national identifications.

Writing of the importance of blood in the history of Western cultures, Michel Foucault observed that blood has constituted one of the "fundamental values."[7] He explains that "power spoke *through* blood: the honor of war, the fear of famine, the triumph of death, the sovereign with his sword, executioners, and tortures; blood was *a reality with a symbolic function*."[8] Although this symbolism has transformed into an "analytics of sexuality" in Foucault's work, blood continues to act as a defining trope of identity and power in cultures around the world. It repeatedly distinguishes between the in-group and the out-group, the stranger from the kin, the illicit from the pure. Blood is metaphorically appropriated as both a marker of life and of death; a symbol of good health and perilous disease. It delineates levels of citizenship, status, relationships, and identities.

Among the more recent metaphors to flow from blood discourses is the notion of "the gift." Since World War II, the altruistic act of blood donation has come to be viewed as a common site of community building, something that benefits not only individuals, but the community as a whole. One act of giving blood can save up to six people at a time and costs nothing on the part of the donor. As noted in the first chapter, blood donation is a performative act of civic engagement and nation building. Citizens are instilled with the notion that they should regularly give blood and repeat acts of selflessness to help others survive. The sacrificial ritual performatively reproduces national identifications among those in the polity. When faced with blood that may be "tainted" or "poison," however, the act of altruism is subverted and blood is no longer regarded as a gift of life, but a vehicle of demise. Far from being an isolated problem that confronts individuals, compromising the safety of the blood supply compromises the security of the nation-state.

This chapter examines the relationship between citizenship, blood donation, and sexuality by exploring how queer blood is rhetorically articulated as deleteriously impure. It is worth repeating that such constructions are impossibly complex, even if there is a strong temptation to label them as simple prejudices. The emphasis on civic identity makes the ban especially complicated because it conjures up discourses of civil rights, even when donating blood is not a right in the traditional sense. Despite the fact that giving blood is not ascribed the status of a civil right, it is almost universally linked to a symbolics of kinship and group belonging. In this sense, blood is closely related to citizenship, even if that relationship is not explicitly written into law. Following Lauren Berlant, citizenship here is not meant in mere legal terms but instead in "the experiential, vernacular context in which people customarily understand their relation to state power and social membership."[9] Chantal Mouffe reminds us that "the way we define citizenship is intimately linked to the kind of society and political community we want."[10] Or, of course, what we don't want. Blood is an implicit cultural metaphor that materializes in specific instances to substantiate claims to civic identity. In our everyday performances of citizenship, there are few occasions when people are hailed to express their commitments to the polity.[11] The explicit avowal of civic identity in the ritual space is an exception to this quiet understanding, performing an illocutionary function that brings identity to fruition in the practice of giving blood. Danielle Allen has powerfully contended that sacrifice "is the only act that might convince others to abandon legal for ethical forms of reciprocity and to seek suppler means than strict barter to preserve autonomy."[12] Blood is representative of community and donation a marker of stranger relationality that engenders trust.

Queer bodies are not merely cast outside the polity under the logic of the blood ban. Like the first John Doe, the containment and marginalization of queer bodies is central to securing a normative center for others enacting their privileges. Men who have sex with other men are positioned within this cultural framework as the embodiment of a distorted citizenship—they are situated as an abjected stranger in the culture they inhabit. They are trapped between the ideals of the performative nature of citizenship as pure and the reductive positioning of queer identities as contagions. To be clear, the challenge here is not to examine how queer men are merely implicated as "foreign." Nor should we believe that all men who have sex with men are easily oppressed as secondhand citizens. The struggle in the rhetoric of the blood ban is to pinpoint the locations in which these two epistemological notions, that of the citizen and that of the foreigner (stranger, queer), are articulated simultaneously through the rhetorical trope of blood. When the Canadian government charged John Doe with negligent misrepresentation, they failed to take into account that queer bodies are always already positioned as negligent, continually maligned as a misrepresentation of that which is deemed normal by institutional power structures.

The materialization of civic identity as it is articulated with nation and queerness through blood donation will be examined in several steps. First, Foucault's conception of bio-power is revisited in relation to the tropes of reproduction and sacrifice. The tropes of sacrifice and reproduction engender a discourse that imagines a communal identity that is constantly positioned in a state of becoming. However, being articulated with AIDS, men who have sex with men invert the idea of stabilizing and building communal identity. When this notion of identity in a state of becoming is articulated with a notion of identity that is constructed as being in a literal and performative state of decay, queer men are the imagined, abject other who pose a threat to the purity of the nation. This convoluted discourse is grounded at the end of the chapter with a close reading of the question, "are you a male who has had sexual contact with another male, even once, since 1977?" Queer men are realized as both inside and outside the system; as impure separatists and polluted assimilationists; as rhetorically contained but ubiquitously promiscuous. In marginalizing queer bodies, the state concurrently produces a normative citizen ideal to reproduce national identity.

ENACTING BIO-POWER / ENABLING CITIZENSHIP

The last several centuries have witnessed a substantial change in how states regulate populations and exert influence over modes of reproduction. As democratic cultures developed, rituals that were once used to "restore the corporal integrity of the monarch" were replaced with therapeutic devices that could be employed to monitor contagions.[13] Novel methods of disciplining bodies materialized in various establishments including medicine, education, and the law to "rationalize" problems posed by deviant populations and implement solutions for managing their presence. Foucault called the ability of the state to utilize expert discourses for the purpose of regulating bodies "bio-power" or "bio-politics." These new and evolving forms of knowledge included everything from the rhetorical appropriation of statistics to the discursive development of lifestyles and a normatively driven ethics of sound health.[14]

Foucault identified two intertwined poles of development that were especially significant for the implementation of bodies working in the service of the state. The first of these strategies was the configuring of bodies as "machines." The state focused on the usefulness and docility of the body for economic and cultural gain, with docility being defined as that which is "subjected, used, transformed and improved."[15] Novel (and often sinister) modes of bodily control were developed in prisons, hospitals, and military institutions to recalibrate relations of power.[16] State discourses were able to fashion that docility, and in doing so reinforced the second element of bio-power, that of the body as a biological entity, being concerned with the tenants of health and reproduction.[17] Far from being two disparate poles of development, these discursive strategies served to reinforce one another and further the state's ability to control and discipline bodies.

Bio-power is embraced by agencies of control to reinforce the power of normative behavior in citizens. This normalization is almost always sculpted in a manner that favors a seemingly natural positioning of heterosexuality. Michael Warner and Lauren Berlant have captured the nature of such normalization well, famously asserting: "Heteronormativity is more than ideology, or prejudice, or phobia against gays and lesbians; it is produced in almost every aspect of the forms of and arrangements of social life: nationality, the state, and the law; commerce; medicine; education; plus the conventions and affects of narrativity, romance, and other protected spaces of culture. It is hard to see these fields as heteronormative because the sexual culture straight people inhabit is so diffuse, a mix of languages they are just developing with notions of sexuality so ancient that their material conditions feel hardwired into personhood."[18] The imperative suggested here is to search out and expose those sites that reinforce debilitating normative behaviors and stunt their power to discipline sexual "deviants," relegating them to a position that is lesser than "ordinary" citizens.

Reflecting on the complex materialization of sexual identities, Judith Butler has pondered "to what extent do *regulatory practices* of gender formation and division constitute identity, the internal coherence of the subject, indeed, the self-identical status of the person?"[19] Butler contends that heterosexuality becomes naturalized through normative performances, by "setting up certain illusions of continuity between sex, gender, and desire."[20] Far from being a simple form of self-expression, performativity stresses an ambiguous reiterative power of discourse to produce and regulate subjects.[21] For Butler, lesbian and gay identifications foster the potential for subverting this signifying process by exposing the limitations of mimesis. In divulging the imitation that performances attempt to approximate, a space is produced between intervals where normative heterosexuality is exposed to subversion. In other words, naturalized performances are actually unstable sites of identity production, continually prone to insurrection.[22]

The current blood ban that has been implemented against men who have sex with other men is one site to begin scrutinizing the processes of normalized citizenship. It is the sexual act that is the focus of factions wishing to contain queer bodies. The blood ban offers us a specific ritual, a place where the reiterative performances Butler speaks of transpire on a daily basis. In posing the question, "are you a male who has had sexual contact with another male, even once, since 1977," there is more than mere exclusion transpiring. The very materialization of citizenship is being policed. If we agree with Foucault's contention that "where there is power, there is resistance," then focusing on this diabolical question highlights the very potential to disrupt the biopower of the state that subjects queer men as pollutants. The oversimplification that is constituted in this question is not only a source of discrimination and normalization, but a site of contestation and illumination. Queer bodies are positioned not as reproducing in their reiteration, but as inciting decay as they attempt to perform acts of civic identity.

Prior to exploring how queer bodies are situated as destructive, it is productive to scrutinize the ways they are rhetorically postured in opposition to notions of the "good citizen" valorized by the state. To accomplish this goal, the following sections will survey two key elements of bio-power. First, the reproductive nature of civic performance and national kinship as envisioned by the state are investigated. Following analysis of that trope, we can turn next to an examination of how sacrifice comes to stand in for the docility of bodies working in the favor of the nation-state. These rhetorical manifestations of bio-power are not wholly disparate and have only been separated for analytic clarity. In fact, a complex relationship exists between the tropes of the reproductive and sacrificial citizen. This convoluted and intertwined association delimits the foundational assumptions inherent in the state's understanding of sexuality and citizenship, forging a misguided notion of queer identities and their relation to larger cultural forms.

THE TROPE OF REPRODUCTIVE CITIZENSHIP

Despite the conflicting metaphors associated with blood (life/death; health/disease), "the juice of life" is almost universally viewed as a marker of kinship lines. One needs only to glance at the ways blood is used to describe relational affiliations to ascertain this significance. We have "bloodlines," "blood relatives," and "blood brothers," among other markers of association. If too closely related by blood, contemporary legal systems often prohibit marriage.[23] Much of the Judeo-Christian Bible deals explicitly with blood and its significant relationship to kinship. Substantial portions of books such as Leviticus inscribe precise rules for defining the relationship between blood and kinship. Not coincidentally, ties to blood in such texts are also where readers are often confronted with the taboo of homosexuality. Homosexual acts inherently cut off the kinship relationship and thus were deemed a dangerous practice associated with idol worship in a world where children were cultural markers of economic and social import.[24]

While understandings of blood have evolved significantly over thousands of years, the symbolic import of blood has been remarkably persistent. In the United States blood has been a particularly important trope of identification. The anthropologist David Schneider has argued that blood is the defining trope of the American character, emphasizing that a "blood relationship is a relationship of identity."[25] Nations, he explains, are structured in the same manner as kinships, with certain relations being constructed as more pure than others.[26] This wholesomeness is especially significant in the imagined kinship of national identity because kinship is not necessarily always already heterosexual.[27] Blood provides "that combination of substance and code for conduct which those who share that red stuff, the blood relatives, should have. In one sense its meaning is reserved to that of substance, in the other it includes both substance and law."[28] Kinship relationships, however, cannot afford to be static entities. They are dependent on the reproduction of citizens in order to carry on the bloodlines of a community. M. Jacqui Alexander reminds readers that the nation has long been conceived as heterosexual, "since biology and reproduction are at the heart of its impulse."[29] Without the proliferation of kin, there is no labor force to produce goods, no military to protect national boundaries, and no populace to ensure the well-being and longevity of state factions. As such, being a "good citizen" is often placed in opposition to those identities that "choose" not to reproduce, as they inherently work against the proliferation of the state. Various sexual practices are poised as being against the "divine order" that helps to sustain the nation. Indeed, some authors have observed that people who invoked such vices "lacked either moral sense or civil responsibility," because they were acting against population propagation.[30]

Certainly, the debates over gay marriage have circulated around the affiliation between and conflation of kinship and citizenship.[31] A common argument against such unions foresees the end of the nation-state if gay relationships are legally sanctioned. These views are clearly supported in an array of cultural institutions ranging from various religious sects to legal entities such as the Supreme Court. As a historical example, in 1986 the U.S. Supreme Court upheld the states' right to prosecute people for committing sodomy in the landmark case *Bowers v. Hardwick.* Calling arguments that guarantee a person's right to privacy "at best, facetious," Justice Byron White asserted in the majority opinion that the defense, representing two gay men who had violated Georgia's sodomy law, had failed to produce the proof necessary to win because ties to procreation were not evident. He asserted that "no connection between family, marriage, or procreation on the one hand and homosexual activity on the other" had been demonstrated.[32] Even after the Court struck down state sodomy laws in the summer of 2003, they chose to focus on individual privacy rights as their determining factor for decision, not moral, communal, or public worth.

The regulation of bodies and fluids in the name of national kinship is further illustrated by the history of states managing the blood of minority populations. Conceptualizing minorities as threats to the reproductive nature of the social body by employing blood as a trope of danger has been a common practice throughout history. Various cultures have established complex myths concerning blood and its relationship to citizens and national character.[33] It is a strategic rhetoric utilized to sustain political hierarchies and discipline various cultural identities. More often than not, blood is constructed in a manner that segregates those who are "pure" from those who "pollute."

Perhaps the most famous example of contemporary blood purification laws transpired in Nazi Germany. The Germans employed science, law, and numerous other cultural forms to stigmatize Jewish people, arguing that their blood was impure and animalistic. In an effort to deal with the "Jewish question," Hitler passed the Nuremberg Laws in September 1935 to delineate differences between German and Jewish citizens. In an attempt to purify kinship lineages, the laws disallowed marriages between Jews and "citizens of German or kindred blood." In addition, it also forbade sexual relations outside of marriage and outlawed the hiring of female Germans as domestic servants to Jews.

Interestingly, it was the Law for the Protection of German Blood, not the Reich Citizenship Law, that disallowed Jewish people from flying the national colors.[34] Section 4 of the act proclaimed that "Jews are forbidden to display the Reich and national flag or the national colors." However, the code also stated that "they are permitted to display the Jewish colors. The exercise of this right is protected by the State."[35] The punishment for misrepresenting the national colors constituted grounds for incarceration up to a year and a monetary fine.[36] There is a complex network of state institutions permeating the ideas at work here. Not only is blood associated with the family, it carries with it economic implications and symbolic representations of the nation. Conversely, the Blood Protection Act was also a method of making visible a substantial portion of the population for state regulation. Hitler permitted Jewish people to fly their "colors" not because of a momentary expression of altruism, but because the blood of the Jews constituted for him a collective kinship, a race. Giving permission to fly the flag allowed the Nazis an opportunity to render visible the people they wished to persecute.

In addition to legal means, the Nazis also employed the voice of science to propagate their ideology of racial purity. German scientists experimented with the idea that blood types could be used as markers among various racial groups, with Aryans, of course, being blood-type A. This falsified classification schema had terrifying consequences, allowing German officials to determine who was, and was not, an authentic member of the state.[37] Despite the seeming ontological groundings this might have produced, blood remained a powerful performative symbol. Hitler reserved the right to grant "clemency" to those whom he judged to "look and act like a person of 'German blood,'" whatever that might have meant.[38] The externalization of blood as a marker of identity in this example draws attention to the performative nature of kinship and the rhetorical manifestations of purity and pollution.

This performative element of national kinship was especially pronounced for extremists of race theory who expressed anxieties about mixing Jewish and German blood. Miscegenation was something to be feared because it helped promote revolution. People who were partially Jewish and partially Aryan were envisioned as dangerous because their blood supposedly equipped them with the "deviousness" of the Jew and the "skill" of the Aryan.[39] Of course, there are analogies to be made between bisexuality and the person of mixed blood feared by the Nazi. It was the boundary crosser that was most to be feared, the one not easily constrained by labels devised by the powers-that-be. Indeed, the bisexual is one who is constantly in danger of entering into the state of decay, but not decomposing alone. The bisexual has the power to draw the imagined heterosexual nation into that state with him as he crosses back over the sexual boundary.[40]

Further, the stereotype that Jews were a threat to children (long preceding Hitler) also reinforced the idea of danger to the kinship lines. Some scholars have found close parallels between the discourses that have incriminated Jewish people and gays and lesbians. Like the stereotype of gay men and lesbians being pedophiles, Jews were falsely posited as physical threats to children, portrayed as killing Christian youth and utilizing their blood to make matzos and cure hemorrhoids.[41] The clear allusion to pure blood being "out of place" to cure hemorrhoids links the imagined sexual prowess of the minorities to their very nature.

It would be remiss to think that narratives involving pure blood were isolated to Nazi Germany. America has a long-standing history of propagating the myth of "pure races." From the arrival of the Irish to the racial "threat" of African Americans, the United States has enforced a discourse of national purity through the myth of sanitized and segregated blood. Noting the importance of national understandings of blood, Ann Laura Stoler comments that "science and medicine may have fueled the re-emergence of the beliefs in blood, but so did nationalist discourse in which a folk theory of contamination based on cultural contagions, not biological taintings, distinguished true members of the body politic from those who were not."[42] The blood of the other has perpetually enabled "normal" citizens to articulate their identities with the culturally sanitized images of the nation-state that circulated in popular discourses of nationalism.

For several decades, transfusing the blood of an African American into a white person without his or her knowledge was a misdemeanor in several states.[43] Such laws stemmed from acts that sought to prevent interracial marriages. As matrimony has long been viewed as the institution that sustains the social order of the state, these laws were designed to regulate kinships and heirs. Although it is often used to describe blood laws, the term "miscegenation" has explicit sexual connotations, albeit racist ones.[44] The term itself was used to produce a "natural" order of things, one that could reinforce structures that have been used to culturally and economically disadvantage African Americans for centuries.

Ironically, it was an African American doctor named Charles Drew who founded the first blood bank in New York in 1941. Despite his work, entities such as the armed forces prohibited the acceptance of blood donations from black citizens. The blood center in the nation's capital was eventually renamed after Drew, but he was among those initially prohibited from donating there. After protests that called the policies prejudiced, the American Red Cross decided to start accepting donations from African Americans, but established rules that kept fluids donated by black Americans segregated from those of whites. Some conservative detractors who supported segregation at the time called the new compromise a "liberal" policy.[45]

Since that time, discourses surrounding blood have continued to develop not only in relation to themes of segregation, but at times, assimilation. The notion of a monolithic blood that is not constrained by the divergence created by the races seems to be a continual part of our culture. Critiquing a *Time* magazine cover that projected the future of American racial identity, Warner and Berlant have concluded that "the nation will become a happy racial mono-culture made up of 'one mixed blood.'"[46] This should not come as a surprise, seeing that national character often trumps images of varying identities.[47]

Clearly, there are important cultural, political, and social differences among the histories of Jewish people, African Americans, and queers (though, many people do occupy all of these identity categories). What remains parallel in their narratives is the degree to which their blood, and their identity, is always signified as more outrageous and dangerous than that of the majority group. Just as a quarter of Jewish blood was more powerful than three-quarters of Aryan blood, and just as "one drop" of black blood was enough to rhetorically contaminate a white body, a minute amount of queer blood (if any) is needed to subvert the reproductive nature of the community. In the discourse of the twentieth century, "one drop" of blood is not very far apart from "one time since 1977."

In this section the bio-political nature of blood as a reproductive force of national kinship identities has been briefly traced. However, along with reproduction, there is a second trope of citizenship valorized by the nation-state and continually reinforced in the rhetoric of the blood ban. The conception of the "sacrifice," that which is done in the service of others and with no personal gain, is a theme that surfaces time and again through state discourses.

THE TROPE OF SACRIFICIAL CITIZENSHIP

Blood donation is perhaps one of the most important forms of cultural sacrifice available to citizens. Not only does it carry with it enormous symbolic import, but it is a ritual that is made readily accessible for people to enact. Donations are regarded as transmutable acts that most citizens can perform, because they cost nothing, are barely time consuming, and can be done in any number of locations. For most Americans, blood donation transcends all partisan politics, perhaps being described in Robert Bellah's words as a "politics of the nation."[48] Briefly, the necessity of dissociating sacrifice from monetary impurities will be revisited. Sanitized from the discursive structure of economics, blood sacrifice can function as a metaphor of national purity.

The sacrificial nature of blood donation is dependent on its necessity to be constructed free of economic implications. The presumptively positive positioning of this exchange as purely altruistic can be traced directly to the publication of Richard Titmuss's 1970 text, *The Gift Relationship*. Here, Titmuss argued that how people understand and relate to cultural conceptions of blood and donation directly influences the safety of the blood supply.[49] Those who conceived of blood as a "gift" and not a paid commodity enhanced the chances of a more pure and secure stock. At the time, he claimed that less than 10 percent of all blood came from volunteers, with most being purchased outright or taken from "captive voluntary donors," such as those in the military or in prison.[50] In his estimates, the effects of buying blood were devastating because it recruited populations that were more likely to abuse drugs and carry hepatitis. His study prompted the United States to reexamine their methods of attracting donors and to establish a system that depended strictly on volunteers.

Although Titmuss's study had great influence, some scholars argue that it was at least partially flawed. Thomas Murray, for example, contends that the United States had largely depended on an altruistic system of donation and, contrary to Titmuss, only a small percentage of the blood supply was purchased. Murray found that Americans took very seriously the idea of offering "the gift of life" because it forged stronger communal bonds.[51] Quite simply, helping others makes people feel good. Both literally and symbolically, blood is a "gift" offered to strangers whom the donor will likely never know. When there is the potential for that gift to create harm, it violates the underlying purposes of the cultural metaphor, causing fear and distrust. Donors, it would seem, are cognizant of this implicit social contract.

Equally significant is Murray's assertion that those who do not have a strong feeling of communal inclusion, often because of cultural marginalization, are less likely to give.[52] Much research, especially as it pertains to the early rhetoric of the ban, suggested that gay men were a large portion of the donor pool, and health officials feared they would cripple the national blood supply by losing a large segment of volunteers.[53] Murray again suggests otherwise, finding "no evidence that gay men were more likely to be donors than other people prior to 1983."[54] This assertion complicates the suggestion that those who generally feel excluded from the community are reluctant to give. Gay men were not *more* likely to donate, but seemingly not *less* likely, either. There remains room to believe that those who have confidence in the system and wish to be included in its fabric might attempt to make the sacrifice. The ritual act may be a personal testimony that people who are omitted find small ways to place themselves in communities that are not always supportive of their identities.[55] Or, there may be layers of exclusion that necessitate more scrutiny from public health officials.

Economic dissociation is a central component of the fantasy of blood sacrifice. Equally significant is the rhetorical space that has been occupied by blood as a cultural marker in American life. As a metaphor, the imagery of sacrificed blood has long been a constitutive force of American identity. It has been present in both conservative and progressive discourses, from the American Revolution to the Second Iraq War. Indeed, some have even used blood sacrifice to connect the American Revolution to the Iraq War.[56] The imagery of sacrificed blood has repeatedly substantiated notions of progress in the American psyche, producing communities that can strive toward the ideals of civic life. Following the church bombing that killed four children in Alabama, for example, the Reverend Martin Luther King Jr. beseeched Americans to convert the senseless crime into a sacrificial discourse emphasizing renewal. He implored his audience, "The innocent blood of these little girls may well serve as the redemptive force that will bring new light into this dark city. . . . The spilt blood of these innocent girls may cause the whole citizenry of Birmingham to transform the negative extremes of a dark past into the positive extremes of a bright future."[57] Savage murder, while initiating unfathomable loss, can be recast as communal sacrifice that provides a catalyst for moral evolution.

The degree to which sacrifice gets woven into national discourses should not be underestimated. Carolyn Marvin and David Ingle have proposed that nationalism is a "civil religion" that depends on the sacrifice of citizens to reinvigorate and reproduce national identity. This faith in the nation is continually reworked in the "stories, images, rites and legal codes of national culture."[58] Just as Abraham was willing to sacrifice his son Isaac to illustrate his pure relationship with God, blood sacrifice in war and in peace operates by purifying the bond between citizens and community.[59] In many ways, this affiliation is rhetorically parallel to the relationship between followers and their religion. It is the memory of the blood sacrifice, in religion or nationalism, which brings the community together. Blood may symbolize the essence of the living, but is simultaneously "associated with pain, injury, and the mystery of death."[60] It is for this reason, then, that the American flag represents freedom to live as one wishes but is fashioned in part using the color red as a representation of bloodshed by soldiers in the Revolutionary War. Bloodlines of the living are connected directly to the bloodlines of the dead.

Kinship connections between the living and the sacrificed dead carry especially significant cultural capital during times of national crisis. When boundaries are being violated and hierarchies blurred, citizens look to suture tears in the social fabric with sacrifices that rhetorically heal rifts. In short, by giving a part of themselves citizens are able to nurture the whole. When no overt public sacrifice is demanded of citizens (which has consistently been the case in regard to the Iraq War), the cause is seen as more corrupt or impure.[61] It is little wonder that the Second World War has been heralded constantly as the "Good War" and the conflict that gave rise to what is frequently referred to as America's "Greatest Generation." Even conscientious objectors to World War II have been remembered in relation to the sacrifice they offered to the country. As the advertising for one PBS special read, "Like combat soldiers, many conscientious objectors were willing to sacrifice themselves for their country. However, they were simply unwilling to kill for it."[62] The centrality of sacrifice to American democracy is especially noteworthy here, as it suggests that blood need not be shed to contribute to the national efforts. However, it is difficult to escape the entrenched imagery of blood sacrifice because the contentious objectors are imagined in direct opposition to slain soldiers.

There are bountiful historical examples of sacrifice and kinship being connected during times of war, but World War II is especially fruitful. Spencie Love described the testimonials of officers who urged citizens to give blood in order to reproduce the ideal of the able-bodied American soldier. Commanding General Jacob L. Devers implored donors by invoking images of soldiers in the field: "When your blood flows into the veins of a wounded soldier, the soldier knows it is more than medicine for his body. It is a part of you that you are giving to help keep him alive. The psychological effect is tremendous . . . Your frequent donation of blood will give them the right they so richly deserve—to live."[63] The relationship is reciprocal in the nature of the sacrifice it is calling for. The soldier is defending the citizen's rights. If she or he can be saved by citizens, they are inherently doing their part to protect the boundaries of the nation and ensure the country's freedom. Not surprisingly, scholars such as Foucault were especially drawn to images of the military to describe the soldier as the docile machine working in favor of the state. When considered in relation to blood and kinship, this docility is especially striking, for soldiers literally protect the national borders. They place themselves in harm's way, and in many senses come to represent the physical manifesta-tion of the "blood sacrifice." In a very religious sense, they die so that the kin (state, nation) may live on.

It is perhaps for this reason that the "gays in the military" debate has caused such a stir. It is in this debate that we see a strong mix between who is embod-ied as both the symbol of health and the representation of a more "purified" sacrifice. Many allusions in the gays in the military debate circulate around the idea of keeping quarters and showers free of contagions, of literally protecting the possibility of permeating the body. The sacrifice should be pure; allowing gays and lesbians into the military violates that pure relationship, those sacri-ficial bonds between soldiers. The attention to physical perfection and clean-liness has been a historically important feature of ritual in a number of reli-gions and cultures.[64] By keeping those in the ritual pure, a closer union to God and country is fostered.

The issue of HIV and AIDS plays an important role in the gays in the mili-tary debate. In the early 1990s male members of the armed forces most fre-quently cited the fear of catching AIDS as a major reason for denying gay people the right to serve.[65] Other studies of police and firemen who work with openly gay men seemed to produce a similar anxiety concerning HIV.[66] Some public opinion polls found that the spread of HIV was seen as one of the primary reasons that people wanted to exclude gays and lesbians, but shar-ing facilities and quarters was always a larger issue.[67]

It is important to note, however, that opinions on issues relating to national sacrifice are historically discriminatory. When the military was racially inte-grated in the 1940s a number of Americans were opposed to it. Polls in 1948 found that upward of 63 percent of Americans were not in favor of mak-ing the armed forces a desegregated institution.[68] As the public feared, when integration in one sphere transpired, it did in others as well. When the bod-ies of African Americans were included, so were their voices in the fabric of the national culture. If they could die for their country, if they provided the blood sacrifice, then they could demand rights. To include gay men and lesbi-ans in the military, then, does not so much give them the right to die for their country so much as it gives them the right to live in it. Several political fac-tions have attempted to argue that focusing on similarities between gays in the military and racial integration are too divergent for comparison. For example, the National Defense Research Institute divided the demographic groups by a number of traits that distinguish the discourses. Among other characteristics of the debate, they focused on everything from the immoral nature of homo-sexuality to budget constraints.

But the most telling of all their arguments that can be linked directly to

the docility factor in sacrificial narratives lies in their final justification for exclusion. In their words, "There is no sense that the change would serve any legitimate need of the military."[69] This particular tenant of their report is revealing. There are strong parallels to the blood ban here, in that the degree
to which gays and lesbians *want* to serve is discounted. The U.S. military had
nothing to gain from allowing gays and lesbians to serve, so alleviating stigma
was seemingly unnecessary. More recently, the man who composed the "don't
ask, don't tell" policy that prohibits gays and lesbians from serving wrote that
the ban should be lifted if the draft is ever reinstated.[70] This would ensure that
heterosexuals could not claim they were gay to avoid war. He does, however,
admit that this would not be a complete repudiation of the policy. As soon as
the war was completed, all information collected could be used against people
who "came out" or were "discovered" to be gay.

While there have been arguments linking queer identities to AIDS (e.g.,
the fear of tainted blood splattering on other soldiers on the battlefield) in
order to justify exclusion, it is certainly not the only line of argumentation advanced by the armed forces. Rather than debate issues of disease that would be
difficult to support, the military focused on more psychological and ritualistic
arguments concerning omissions. In particular, the military seemed preoccupied with membership "morale" and "cohesion." Homosexuality disrupts cohesion, being understood not as something that builds community, but something that destroys collective bonds. It renders impotent the idea of the blood
sacrifice, the notion that one is protecting the purity of the American state.
The image of the diseased and infected body regularly positions gays and lesbians as both lesser citizens and a threat. When we think of the military body,
it is not feeble and heterogeneous but instead uniform and erect.[71]

Consistently, gay people in the military are linked to disorder and chaos.
The National Defense Research Institute writes that militaries are based on
a "formal, hierarchical, and rule driven structure, which values efficiency,
predictability, and stability in operations. This structure is supported and
reinforced by organizational and participant cultures that are conservative,
rooted in history and tradition, based on group loyalty and conformity, and
oriented toward obedience to superiors."[72] Thomas Yingling's assertion that
homosexuality is always that point at which everything seems to have got-
ten out of hand is relevant here.[73] Gays and lesbians are judged as people who
uniformly lack formality, violate hierarchies, uproot history, defile tradition,
and ignore superiors. They have the ability to produce pure chaos, and in the
military such disorder is where lives will surely be lost. This disruption of cohesion, this fear of the stranger in the barricades, gives rise to the idea that gay
people preclude states of becoming. In the eyes of the state, they are articulated as an impending signature of death.

The trope of sacrifice sustains the trope of reproduction, thus perpetuating the kinship of national identity. Good citizens do what they can do to reproduce and sacrifice when necessary. Unfortunately, it is usually for the state to decide when that sacrifice is and is not allowed. In the next section it will become increasingly evident that men who have sex with other men are regarded as markers of death, occupying identities that endanger civic life.

IN A STATE OF NON-BECOMING

The idea of a performative citizenry that constantly reproduces in order to sustain the community stands in sharp contrast to the fears that are associated with AIDS and queer men. In the eyes of the state, performative acts reinforcing the order of things are impaired by homosexuality. A man who has had sex with another man is rhetorically enacted as a figure of chaotic embodiment, the so-called sexual deviant. Articulated with AIDS, homosexuality takes on new powers and presents more horrific threats. So pungent is homosexual ontology that it takes but one act of intimacy since 1977 to compromise the safety of the kin and the security of the nation—indefinitely. In this manner, the body politic needs to be protected from the virus that is spreading from within. The sexual act is framed not as a momentary happening, but a certain nexus of temporal horizons, "the condensation of an iterability that exceeds the moment it occasions."[74] This excessiveness and its seemingly hazardous by-products must be contained to assure national security.

Of course, it is impossible to address the paranoia of the singular act without discussing the profound impact that AIDS has had on our culture. The expansiveness of AIDS has given rise to a new set of complications for communal conceptions of citizenship and the role of the individual in the body politic. In contrast to the continual state of becoming that is reinforced by modes of reproduction, AIDS has signaled the loss of the body, the implosion of identity, and the stagnation of development. With the rise of AIDS discourses we have, in Yingling's words, an "alienation from a body that no longer seems to house a subject," one that foregrounds "the impossibility of speaking the condition of loss being written into (and onto) the body . . . the whole problem of a disappearing body, of a body quite literally shitting itself away."[75] The apocalyptic implosion of the citizen subject signals a loss of bio-political control and the reproduction of civic actors and sacrificial bodies. Even as we acknowledge the progress made against HIV, in the cultural imaginary AIDS is still largely conceived as prompting disintegration.

A body no longer in a state of becoming stands in sharp contrast to the usual notions of identity that have been embraced by scores of academic scholars. The presupposition that we are constantly in a state of becoming is offset by a constellation of discourses emphasizing waste and erosion. Throughout much of the epidemic, a body with AIDS has been rhetorically constructed in the manner Yingling described, not in a state of "avoiding decay," but of literally decomposing. The resuscitation of identifications is persistently situated as being stifled by the progressive onset of disease. Although HIV/AIDS is now widely regarded as "manageable," medical and cultural discourses continue to emphasize a focus on forestalling decay and mobilizing stability. Regardless, the blood ban perpetuates these logics of dissolution, insisting that all queer men are potential agents of death.

Discursively, there have been great strides taken to distance the heterosexual state from the dangers that are associated with AIDS. Although AIDS was once largely viewed as an American disease (because of the visibility first given to white gay American men), there have been significant attempts to shift the focus to the problem of AIDS in other nations, forging it into a "foreign" disease. Normative heterosexual citizenship, for example, has consistently been recuperated by media labels such as "African AIDS."[76] Displacing heterosexual AIDS to another continent has alleviated fears among heterosexual Americans about the threat of infection, allowing them to continue sexual practices that seemingly do not implicate their identities. By inserting racist notions of black men in Africa as dangerous and culturally uneducated, Western states can reassure its populations that "African AIDS" spreads more quickly and terribly. By blaming culture as the mark of impurity, the state can draw attention away from the fact it withholds money for drugs and other programs to prevent disease.[77]

National discourses not only distance the threat of AIDS as a foreign entity rhetorically, they also seek to establish the idea that AIDS can be subsumed by invoking laws that speciously claim to protect the nation's boundaries. In 1987 Congress passed legislation requiring all people immigrating to the United States, or requesting visas, to be HIV-negative. At the time the bill was passed the United States had the highest rates of HIV/AIDS cases in the world. There was a false sense of security promoted in the bill. If Congress could simply seal off the boundaries of the nation, the impending threat would be prohibited and eventually the menace of AIDS would fade away.[78] Quite literally, the foreigner came to be the ultimate scapegoat in the fight against HIV.[79] It is certainly no coincidence that countries such as Kenya and Zaire, nations that were distant and located in the African continent, came to be among the most prominently featured as potential points of origin for the HIV virus. Just as lawmakers have worked hard to position ideas and practices that threaten democracy outside national boundaries (communism, terrorism), so too have they attempted to isolate AIDS apart from the national imaginary of everyday life.[80] However, such images were far from consistent in their form or content, as contradictory notions of AIDS were often invoked. While heterosexual people of color outside the nation were continually being exposed to HIV, only gay white men were supposedly afflicted with the virus domestically.[81]

"Men who have sex with other men" share an affinity with this presumed foreignness when situated in relation to the blood ban. If state powers can simply prevent these men from donating blood, then the heterosexual populace can take some refuge that they are not only safe, but always already more pure than their queer counterparts. The sentiment that heterosexuals can have numerous partners, donate blood, and still save the lives of others is protected if the nation can impart intimate pictures of gay and bisexual men as threats.[82]

This notion of a decaying and contaminated identity is not exclusive to debates surrounding the blood ban. A number of issues involving sexuality have been structured around the trope of the diseased body, especially in relation to nationalistic discourses. Returning to the "gays in the military" debate, for example, there is a clear reinforcement of impurity metaphors emphasizing the destabilization of the nation. Judith Butler has persuasively argued that homosexuality becomes rhetorically figured on the model of AIDS and communicated along the lines of a contagion throughout the "gays in the military" debate.[83] She explains that "within contemporary military discourse, the taboo status of homosexuality is intensified by the phobic reduction of homosexual relations to the communication of AIDS, intensifying the sense of homosexual proclamations as contagious acts."[84] This articulation between homosexuality and AIDS inevitably leads to a potent site of discrimination because it "provides only negative structures of identification," as AIDS carries with it substantial powers to produce non-identities and "internalized abjection."[85]

Disciplining sexual identity transpires in many segments of culture, and understanding dominant rhetorics of decay cannot be accomplished without exploring numerous social forms that attempt to formulate and regulate civic identity. May Joseph has elucidated this point, explaining that all people "are constantly impinged on as citizen-subjects, operating between the legal, the cultural, and the political, often in tandem, in our everyday gestures."[86] The materialization of citizenship here transpires not just in transcripted elements of the law, but in all aspects of life. Indeed, few matters of citizenship as they relate to sexuality are contained within a strictly "legal sphere," as many texts (including several concerning LGBT rights) would have us believe.[87] This complex network of institutional influence over sexual citizenship has a long standing in American governmental history. For example, when the state of

Florida released its report, *Homosexuality and Citizenship in Florida,* it framed issues of sexuality as a problem not merely for government, but for "educators, psychiatrists, psychologists, researchers, social workers, law enforcement and judicial officials, and practicing homosexuals themselves."[88] The church and the family are among the other ideological state apparatuses that surface as the report's conspiratorial theme develops. All institutions, public and private, were vulnerable to the dangers associated with homosexuality.

Despite its ever-presence, homosexuality is simultaneously constructed as foreign, with the potential to infect the state and bring harm to "normal" citizens. So, while Florida officials recognized the seeming threat of homosexuality, they claimed "no corner on understanding the history or prognosis of homosexuality."[89] They were, however, "convinced that many facets of homosexual practice as it exists in Florida . . . pose a threat to the health and moral well-being of a sizable portion of our population."[90] In the eyes of the state, homosexuality is foreign, but domestic. It is present everywhere, but without a history or a home. It can be diagnosed, but seemingly without diagnostic methods.

ARTICULATING ABJECTION

Civic identity is not an ontologically based state of being so much as it is a performative reiteration of articulations. Articulation here is meant in the manner that Stuart Hall described it, as "the form of the connection that *can* make a unity of two different elements, under certain conditions," although such linkages are not deterministic and absolute.[91] Lawrence Grossberg adds that articulation is "the production of identity on top of difference....Articulation links this practice to that effect, this text to that meaning, this meaning to that reality, this experience to those politics."[92] Such articulations work on a number of levels that are epistemological, political, and strategic.[93] Moreover, new articulations coming to fruition (such as those explored in the final chapters of this book) are always possible.

Two articulations have already merited particular attention in this study. The first of these involved the problematic, but long-standing association between gay men and AIDS. To regulate blood, the state rhetorically positions the two as indistinguishable. The second articulation is more convoluted in both its focus and its framing. There is a clear articulation of community as constantly in a state of becoming, coupled with homosexual embodiment that is constantly in a state of decay. Each of these subverts the tropes of sacrifice and reproduction central to kinship and community building. State agencies such as the FDA work hard to ensure the populace that social structures are resolutely fortified so that citizens can assume definitive identifications with the nation. The government uses the shadow of the other to constitute a normative citizenship, ensuring the public that their marriages are defended and their blood pure. A specific kind of queer citizen emerges from these articulations, one who is located both inside and outside the political body. This citizen is simultaneously a domestic product and a foreign subject, occupying a position that necessitates perpetual surveillance and control.

While one might ponder why anybody would desire inclusion into such a brutally heterosexist system, it remains a fact that those who occupy marginalized positions often work hard to be included into the fabric of the imagined national identity.[94] Despite strong urges to resist assimilation by some, social movements based on identity, such as the LGBT movement, can strengthen existing nation-states by calling for inclusion. As such, the emergence of identity groups may reinvigorate the nation-state's politics and enlarge its ability to regulate bodies.[95] Goffman suggests that it is those stigmatized individuals who must come to accept themselves as essentially the same as other citizens. However, unlike numerous citizens, men who have sex with other men must frequently and voluntarily withhold from situations in which other citizens would have to proclaim civic acceptance and symbolic unity—as with the blood ritual.[96] Stigmatized people are positioned to "reciprocate naturally with an acceptance" of themselves that the culture has never really offered them in the first place.[97] Indeed, when AIDS was first discovered as a disease that afflicted gay men, it was given little attention. Yingling painfully reminds readers that "the deaths of thousands of homosexual men did not solicit *any* government response for so long in part because homosexual men were not recognized as constituents of the (now infamously phrased) 'general population.'"[98] When they were finally included in such discourses, it was often at the expense of their identities as gay men.

This state of existing between worlds, being articulated as part of the social body and concurrently discarded by it, is reminiscent of Julia Kristeva's conception of the abject. She explains that the abject "is something rejected from which one does not part, from which one does not protect oneself as from an object."[99] The abject is a space in which borders become unclear and matter is seemingly "out of place." The classic examples of such ambiguity are body fluids: puss, excrement, and, of course, blood. When we bleed the border between the inside of the body and the outside is blurred, connection and repulsion exist in tandem. Kristeva writes that "the abject is perverse because it neither gives up nor assumes a prohibition, a rule, or a law; but turns them aside, misleads, corrupts; uses them, takes advantage of them, the better to deny them. It kills in the name of life—a progressive despot."[100]

Kristeva makes only a passing mention of homosexuality in her discussion of the abject in *Powers of Horror*. Fortunately, scholars such as Iris Marion Young have appropriated this notion of "abjection" to examine racism, sexism, and homophobia. She asserts that "homophobia is one of the deepest-held fears of difference precisely because the border between gay and straight is constructed as the most permeable . . . so the only way to defend my identity is to turn away with irrational disgust."[101] Certainly, gays and lesbians are among the most abject of citizens both because of the degree to which they blur gender roles and because they allow for taboo matter to exist "out of place."

Yet the very form of nationalistic social movement discourse, that of being included in the system, forces a reproduction of the rhetorical appeal for the inclusion of queer blood. Indeed, "the sacrificial system of nationalism can be challenged effectively only by those who embrace with still greater commitment alternative sacrificial systems to replace it."[102] In the eyes of the state, queers must accept themselves as essentially the same as others, even if they are being denied privileges afforded to other groups. As Warner argues, there "has always been a close and necessary relation between the cultural form of voluntary association and the cultural norms of expressive individualism."[103] In this sense, donating blood is advanced as being "above" an individual's right to participate in the political sphere. Giving blood is first and foremost concerned with the well-being of another, and the need to protect that person (even when a threat does not exist) trumps a perspective donor's right to partake in the community ritual. In some ways, donating blood during a time of national crisis is very much parallel to speaking out during a national crisis. While everyone usually agrees that people have the right to protest the actions of the state, that freedom is pitted against the fragility of the soldier who is sacrificing her or his body in the name of the nation-state. A distorted form of "involuntary sacrifice" is required of the queer blood donor.

This is certainly the case in the example of John Doe and the Canadian Blood Services mentioned at the start of this chapter. The logic of the state dictates that altruistic tendencies should have encouraged John Doe to understand himself as aiding the community most when he removed himself from the donor pool, not when he offered a contribution. After all, "John Doe" not only connotes the idea of the anonymous, it traditionally constitutes the workings of the everyday man.[104] On occasion people are given the ubiquitous label in order to be protected from state factions in legal battles, but most often when we talk about "any John Doe" or "Jane Doe" on the street, we are contemplating the embodiment of the common citizen. As Richard Dyer has noted, "John Doe" is a symbol of normalization, a telling sign of white masculinity. This masculinity occupies the space of the ordinary, and in some manners, invisibility.[105] When employing the phrase "John Doe," there is an attempt to capture the imagined notion of the conventional individual in the larger social fabric.

The use of "John Doe" in the case of the Canadian blood donation, however, implies something more dangerous than "the everyday citizen." Just as in Dyer's critique of the film *Seven,* the conception "John Doe" is more a representation of the potential hazards of seemingly normal people than of the average guy.[106] This is precisely how the queer citizen is rhetorically molded by advocates of the blood ban. People may appear normal, but underlying these performances are the perils that accompany the queerness of the stranger and their potentially treacherous motives. It is reminiscent of Kristeva's discussion of the stranger in the body politic. As she writes, "Living with the other, with the foreigner, confronts us with the possibility or not of *being an other.*"[107]

Kristeva's words are especially haunting when we rethink the very nature of donation during times of national crisis. A "crisis," quite literally, is a breakdown of meaning. People donated blood in the days following the Oklahoma City Bombing and September 11, not simply because it was an act of altruism, but also because the reiterative performance functions to stabilize identity and forge reidentification with that which is familiar and normal. When confronted with a situation that provides ambiguity and uncertainty, there is little room for tolerance of that which is different. The mere fact that the ARC discarded most of the blood it collected following the September 11 attacks had little to do with why people donated it in the first place. There is a need and a determination to stabilize that which is not stable and re-center our basic understanding of whom we imagine ourselves being. This is why donations usually occur in spaces traditionally understood in relation to the community. Blood drives do not simply take place anywhere. Aside from collection agencies, they are most commonly held in schools, town halls, churches, and other local institutions that are tied to larger social structures. The public performance of blood donation engenders the materialization of civic identity.

Of course, merely lifting the blood ban on queer men will not alleviate the stigma that has been projected onto them. However, forging a policy that focuses on unsafe sex and not on uncertain claims about individual behavior will open a space for rethinking the manner in which "men who have sex with other men" could be introduced. Queer people have long been accused of "contaminating" the cultural and political landscape of the country. It is imperative to seek out those sites that expose the falsity of heterosexual performances and identities as imagined by the state as more pure than others. The blood ban provides one such site of investigation.

"JOHN DOE" AND THE RITUAL OF
REITERATING IDENTITIES

Although it has long been known that AIDS affects people of all races, classes, genders, sexualities, and nationalities, the discourses surrounding the blood ban continually return to the rhetorical appropriation of a "high-risk population" that endangers public health. To erase overt stigmatization, state agencies carefully supplant direct blame by employing disclaimers that purport to discriminate equally across populations. The particular rhetorical strategy that will be examined in this final segment is the question that is posed to people each time they attempt to donate blood, that query being, "are you a male who has had sexual contact with another male, even once, since 1977?" This question presents both a cleansing of sexual identity and an overt homosexual specter; the word "gay" is never mentioned, yet gay sex remains a constant presence. There is an odd conceptual appropriation of the term "queer," one that recognizes the fluid nature of sexuality, all the while disciplining it as an abnormal presence.

This final section will set up the epistemological framework that guides the discursive attitudes authorizing the blood ban. Essential to the deployment of this stigmatization is the creation of knowledge about queer bodies that is outside the reach of the population it is marginalizing. Far from a straightforward discrimination, the strategic use of bio-politics and the positioning of abject citizens is hard work, and in the construction of the queer body, there must be a set of understandings that lie primarily within the realm of state discourses and the agencies that underscore the reproductive needs of the nation. Numerous contradictions surface in the epistemological framework surrounding the question, "are you a male who has had sexual contact with another male, even once, since 1977?" However, these contradictions do not serve to subvert the power of the state. The discursive incongruity established in this question highlights the precise and ubiquitous ways discrimination transpires.[108]

While the FDA's invasive question allows for a degree of self-awareness concerning the body (most people will know if they have engaged in sexual activity), such understandings are not always easily delimited. We need only examine the complications that accompany the term "sex" and its divergent meanings to underscore the problems that surface when employing ambiguous language. The word "sex" has long been a source of debate in communities attempting to resist heteronormative understandings of pleasure and desire often connected to reproduction. Indeed, the term "sex" constitutes something different for any number of people. In the case of a "man who has had sex with another man," it becomes important to ponder how "sex" is being defined by officials at the FDA. Can sex be defined as oral or anal? Does mutual masturbation count as sex? Must penetration occur? If so, what kind of penetration?

The ambiguity of the term, however, is perhaps its greatest power. It forces people who have no access or inclination toward heterosexual sex to answer in the affirmative, or to deny that their sexual experiences are as genuine as their heterosexual counterparts. For gay men, this question functions in a manner that denigrates their identity regardless of the answer they provide. Responding, "yes, I have had sex with another man" separates them from the community and stigmatizes their sexuality. Lying to the state agencies by replying in the negative forcibly removes queer identities by refusing to recognize the contributions that sexual minorities have to offer.

Conversely, the ambiguity of the term "sex" could also position men who have engaged in sexual acts with other men, but who do not consider anything outside of penetration to be real sex, to answer in a manner contrary to the FDA's intents. Numerous cultures, especially those that are hostile to gay and lesbian identity, often disregard anything outside of heterosexual coitus to be sex. So, far from being a term that simply stigmatizes out-of-the-closet gay men, the question also influences "men who have 'sex' with other men" to interpret the question as not pertaining to their sexual activities. As such, it positions a variety of men who might contribute blood to answer "incorrectly."

While the term "sex" may be a source of ambiguity, it is framed by a closed question that forces a definitive reply. Answering "maybe" to "have you had sex with another man" is certainly not permitted and would be immediate grounds for suspicious blood and the suspension of donation privileges. Rather than prescribe an understanding of sex for the person offering the blood donation, the question impels queer men to identify their own understandings of sex and verbalize them. Unlike a number of forums that allow for complex dialogues concerning queer identity and sexuality, however, one is placed in the precarious position of answering "yes" or "no" to the question. There is no room for ambiguity.

The double bind surrounding the question is striking. In the site where self-sacrifice for the community transpires, determining which epistemology to reproduce becomes imperative. Despite all other factors concerning safety and identity, one could reinforce the discursive power the state already maintains over sexual identity by replying "yes," and allowing for further stigmatization. Or, in this place where communal altruism and honesty supersedes all else, a donor could withhold what might be a significant portion of one's identity and answer "no" on the principle that all people be included. This is not meant to imply that the donor is inherently degraded of all self-worth; but the donor is patently positioned to self-discipline. It is, as Sedgwick reminds us, the nature of the discursive closet to punish gays and lesbians not only for being too visible, but for not being visible enough.[109]

This visibility, the need of the state and blood agencies to locate bodies in order to create knowledge about them, is at the very heart of this debate. The question, "are you a male who has had sexual contact with another male, even once, since 1977?" makes this necessity of visibility noticeably transparent. Indeed, bio-politics and the tropes of sacrifice and reproduction are not simply subverted by the person who is being confronted with the questionnaire at blood donation centers. Perhaps the most potent, subtle imagery comes not from the direct information that is being solicited from the person being interviewed, but by the imagined "other" that is projected in the institutional query. Indeed, the phrase, "have you had sex with another man," implicates not only the person being interviewed, but also reveals a third party's presence in the exchange. The "other man" mentioned in the question becomes as epistemologically significant as the rejected donor to the regulatory agencies. Here we have a faceless representation of homosexuality, one that is scientifically formulated and performatively imagined in the ritual of donation. He is the literal and figurative "John Doe" in the eyes of the state, one who walks among the populace as both a stranger and a threat.

The imagined third party in the medical phrase described above is an important rhetorical trope in the discourses that propel the legitimacy of the blood ban. Perhaps more than any other, it is this imagined individual, much like the imagined figure of the AIDS-infested African body, that reveals both the anxieties of disease and the false securities circulated among heterosexual populations. Unlike the imagined victims overseas, however, this "other man" walks invisibly among the populace. The unknown figure is beyond institutional knowledge and concurrently the ontological representation of queer men.

Primarily, the figure of the queer man imagined here is one the state can never know with any degree of measure. When given access to personal information, the ARC and related agencies know nothing more about "the other" man than his figurative representation of the sexual act that transpired. His being is inaccessible to health officials, AIDS tests, and the other regulatory features that ensure the safety of the blood supply. The imagined body becomes a space that is replete with unanswered questions concerning sex and the degree to which this person might not act with the same altruistic intents of the donor with whom he was sexually engaged.

The unknown element of this abject creature stands in sharp contrast to the definitive nature of the remainder of the question. The date "1977" placed at the query's closure acts as an epistemological marker in a manner that the unknown man cannot. For while scientists and government officials are not able to determine with any degree of certainty when the sexual act took place, they can say that having sex since that time constitutes a dangerous threat, a risk violation that was as dangerous prior to AIDS education as it is today. The year 1977 marks a time when that elusive virus started becoming most threatening and hazardous to the well-being of middle America. While state agencies cannot always determine the visibility of the syndrome it-self, they can invoke a method that forces a degree of certainty on to the situation.[110]

This very ambiguity, however, this inability of the state to answer with a degree of epistemological knowledge, is precisely what empowers its contro-versial decision to exclude queer blood. In blood collection there is a continual push to gather the healthiest and purest blood available to those who will reap its benefits. As such, that which can be definitively "known" must act as the most significant identification mechanism for organizations concerned with the collection of blood products. If there is any information concerning do-nors that exists outside the realm of understanding for collectors, it is auto-matically presupposed to be a potential source of imperilment for collection agencies. As a result, the question gives license to agencies to exclude queer donors, as their imagined sexual escapades are rhetorically constructed as more impure and unknown than other members of the polity.

Official discourses, however, always situate themselves in a position of "knowing," even when they claim complete ignorance. Hence, the "other man" in the blood-donor questionnaire occupies a space that allows the state to claim that it is ignorant of queer sexuality and simultaneously becomes a source for representing the known dangers of that sexuality. In the forcible act of excluding queer men from blood donation, the "other man" becomes a metaphorical embodiment of contagion, a site that inverts that space of the altruistic blood gift. Even when seemingly invisible, it is that very absence that allows for the imagination of regulatory regimes to concoct specific under-standings of the queer body.

This epistemological and ontological understanding of sexuality trumps the knowledge that queer men themselves hold about their sexual partners. Al-though men may know who their sexual partners are, what sexual acts trans-pired, and the health of their partners and themselves, this self-awareness is never enough to trump state-sanctioned knowledge. Assertions of self-knowledge have long been trumped publicly by an onslaught of public health officials, religious leaders, and legal and scholarly experts who claim to have a more compelling understanding of queer lives.[111] Knowledge concerning sexual identity has almost always been discarded unless supported by institutional acknowledgment. In the definitive question posed by the FDA, there is no room for explanation, no space to offer individual details concerning sexuality and how it empowers and inhibits civic responsibilities.

The figure of the "other man," then, is a rhetorical site that the state attempts to discredit the volunteer from genuinely comprehending. Rather than be seen as a secure site of interpersonal relations, the epistemological site of sex is represented as a space that is permanently unstable. In this space, there is no reproduction in the service of the state. Concurrently, the very space where the nonreproductive act took place also becomes the site where the important citizen sacrifice is inherently subverted. By not definitively knowing, and hence creating a stable site of understanding, governing factions can marginalize the blood of the abject citizen and use sound, epistemological understandings as the basis for discrimination.

Drawing attention to the indecipherable nature of sexual praxis in the eyes of the state provides ample room for challenging the stifling forces of normativity and narrow understandings of citizenship. It is equally important, however, to examine how constitutive metaphors of decay are given voice in widely circulated narratives associated with the blood ban. Policy makers necessitate cultural discourses that malign queer men, and the memory of the original blood crisis provides that ammunition. Accordingly, the next chapter explores how queer bodies are endowed with an agency to prevent personal and civic decay, but live in denial about the dangers of their own bodies.

3
AIDS Memory, Medicinal Prudence, and the Construction of Social Denial

The HBO movie adaptation of Randy Shilts's book, *And the Band Played On,* features a disastrous meeting held in January 1983. Organized by the Center for Disease Control, the gathering was called to present information supporting policy initiatives to protect the blood supply from infectious agents. In the film, scientists offer data illustrating the direct relationship of blood, infection, and the populations most likely to harbor the elements that eventually cause AIDS. Composed of representatives from organizations and groups most affected by the possibility of implementing donor deferral policies, the meeting included the American Association of Blood Banks, the National Gay Task Force, the American Red Cross, the National Hemophilia Foundation, and the Pharmaceutical Manufacturers Association.[1] Now regarded as "that horrible meeting" by those who were present, the quorum has been remembered as a moment when preventative measures imposed on donated blood could have saved thousands of lives.[2] By all accounts, the CDC's proposed donor deferral policies were trumped by a vocal gay lobby that feared heightened social stigma and by a blood industry unwilling to pay for additional testing measures.

According to the film, the forum was also occasion to one other momentous happening: the unanimous approval of changing the name of the elusive sickness from GRID (Gay Related Immunodeficiency Disease) to AIDS (Acquired Immune Deficiency Syndrome). Regardless of the copious political differences among the representatives present, they all agreed that infections were not isolated to men who engaged in sex with other men. A new name was necessary to underscore the point that the unfolding epidemic was not wreaking havoc solely on gay men. The more accurate acronym was meant to prevent heterosexuals from assuming they could not infect, or be infected, merely because of their sexual orientation.

Despite the dramatic appeal of this made-for-television moment, this particular gathering was not actually where the name of the elusive illness was changed from GRID to AIDS. The label AIDS had been adopted months before at a meeting attended by several of the aforementioned organizations.[3] Yet, in a few fleeting seconds, *And the Band Played On* defined the epidemic by depicting the exact moment when science designated the name of the unfolding catastrophe and gay people stood in their way. Viewers of the "nonfiction" film were offered representations of the scientific logic employed by government officials to combat the initial crisis, but were also made witness to the baffling and short-sighted objections of a gay community that discounted the self-evident conclusions of epidemiology and virology. Like the film's protagonist, Dr. Don Francis, the audience was prompted to witness the birth of AIDS, but with the anxious certainty that this crisis would inevitably tailspin into an unstoppable pandemic. By quickly splicing the arguments of the seemingly irrational gay lobby, the film never gave close attention to the concerns they raised, including fears of increased stigmatization or parallels to U.S. miscegenation laws.[4]

The struggle to narrate the early AIDS crisis has long been marked by a desire to determine who had access to information that could have saved thousands of lives. Not surprisingly, such efforts have found a home in discourses that isolate those who were "innocent victims" from those who "deserved" AIDS.[5] What remains fascinating about this rhetoric, however, is not simply the inclination to assign blame for a notoriously complicated and convoluted catastrophe. More intriguing are the deep contradictions that mark these accusatory discourses and the disparate cultural forms in which they materialize. While it is often presupposed in cultural memory that gay people had an abundant amount of information regarding AIDS, the ban on donated blood was originally (and continues to be) enforced precisely because queer men seemingly did *not* know that they presented a high risk. The ostensible failure of queer donors to recognize the exigency of the situation signaled a dismissal of scientific evidence, a denial of harm that continues to be mediated in the discourses pertaining to contemporary deferral policies.

In her critique of the cultural memory surrounding AIDS, Marita Sturken argues that AIDS representation enabled a discursive rupture because there were "no mainstream conventions for the depiction of homosexuality and because the cinematic tradition of portraying disease is one of victimization."[6] Sturken suggests that fragmented representations offered resistance to oppressive social stereotypes precisely because cultural codes concerning homosexuality were not wholly codified in the social imaginary. In a Foucauldian sense, opportunities for challenging disparaging notions of gay men were always present in the manifold discourses surrounding AIDS. Despite the value of this critique, the potential that competing depictions of queer men have in sustaining oppressive generalizations should not be underestimated. Often, the fact that there are no mainstream conventions does not present a rupture in culture so much as it sutures a hegemonic social cooptation of identity. The entextualization process renders performative understandings of identity more ontologically secured in memory narratives as time progresses, never attaining closure, but providing an illusion of synthesis among incommensurable discourses. Contradicting visions of social bodies are especially suspicious in rhetorics that valorize witnessing (such as science and documentary) because the phenomenological nature of these forms explains away conflicting cultural factors as irrelevant in the face of "real" evidence.[7]

In regards to the public memory of the blood ban, queer men embodied both the hyper masculine and the excessively docile; they are simultaneously represented as a vocal, self-aware lobby, and as among the most undereducated populations afflicted by AIDS. Regardless of the embedded contradictions, this double bind serves to reinforce discriminatory policies, not subvert injurious politics. Underpinning the rhetorical contradiction between awareness and ignorance is the suggestion that information was properly imparted at the epidemic's inception. Examining contemporary accounts of the early crisis, one might assume that science had disseminated the appropriate knowledge to the public and that gay people had simply neglected its warnings. Reflecting on key examples from AIDS history, such as "that horrible meeting" depicted in *And the Band Played On,* it would seem that numerous populations, such as gay men, were well acquainted with the syndrome and its consequences. While some queer citizens seemingly knew of the crisis and did nothing with that knowledge, others, according to the public script, actively disregarded it. Importantly, this is not to say that all queer men as a collective knew nothing about HIV/AIDS as the epidemic unfolded. Rather, in the public memory of AIDS gay men are frequently positioned as flippant while scientists are valorized as knowing that which was essentially unknown.

In this chapter I argue that particular citizens have been endowed with scientific knowledge in texts that document the early AIDS crisis to alleviate government blame for the blood collection catastrophe. Important media texts have been hegemonically inflected with a *medicinal prudence* that recuperates institutional deliberation and its inability to respond to the AIDS crisis. While the previous chapter described the manner in which the process of blood donation materializes an idealized caricature of the average citizen and his or her social obligation to ritually sustain national identity, this chapter explores how specific citizens are bestowed with establishment knowledge to sustain the credibility of dominant structures. While gay men purportedly abandoned science's warnings, two contrasting figures, the maternal transfusion recipient and the hemophiliac, are presented as fully cognizant of AIDS since its inception. In the following pages, texts that construct a narrative about the origins of the blood ban are scrutinized to investigate the constitution of a medicinal prudence that is dependent on, yet strategically divorced from, queer identities. Gay men are positioned to represent the very antithesis of cultural prudence—the embodiment of social denial.

This chapter considers both mainstream media representations and public health rhetorics that detail the contamination of the blood supply. Although outwardly disparate, these discourses are closely intertwined, perpetuating a narrative that advances a particular understanding of queer sex, civic responsibility, and science. Two films based on scientific accounts of the unfolding epidemic, *And the Band Played On* and *Red Gold: The Epic Story of Blood,* are among the cultural artifacts considered. Also under examination are the books on which each of these productions are based, Randy Shilts's *And the Band Played On* and Douglas Starr's *Blood: An Epic History of Medicine and Commerce.* These books bridge the gap between scientific data and popular representations, helping to forge a powerful cultural narrative that posits the queer community against more aware, and hence more pure, citizen bodies.

MEDIATING MEDICINAL PRUDENCE

Despite the numerous historical records detailing the development of AIDS, attempts to educate various populations about its dangers, and early accounts of activist groups such as ACT-UP, there are potentially no archives detailing the implementation of the blood ban.[8] Requests put in to the Center for Disease Control, the Food and Drug Administration, the American Red Cross, the Gay Men's Health Crisis, the National Institute of Health, and the New York Public Library turned up no materials documenting the procedures used to alert blood collection agencies about restrictions, attempts to notify regular gay blood donors, or public displays announcing the plan. No agency claims to house pamphlets, posters, or other materials that encouraged gay men to withhold from giving blood at donation centers or other places of public import. This loss includes records of "that horrible meeting" in 1983.[9]

Of course, discovering there is no archive is never quite as compelling as unearthing an untouched wellspring of materials. This absence of information presents a staggering barrier, as an important epoch of the AIDS epidemic remains hidden and with it significant details concerning education, health awareness, and policy implementation. These unmapped moments, however, have proven valuable for memory scholars such as Barbie Zelizer, who notes that "incompleteness becomes no less compelling when we consider what has been left out of the study of memory by virtue of its being left out of memory itself—the omissions, rearrangements, strategic moments of forgetting."[10] In the realm of collective consciousness, absence structures memory. Information privileged by marginalized groups is often lost in dominant cultural narratives that attempt to suture discursive rifts created by social crises. These absences invite questions about how donor deferral strategies have come to be remembered and the form in which knowledge about the epidemic helps sustain policies adopted against men who have sex with other men in the "interest" of public health. Epidemics, Foucault reminds us, are discursively positioned and appropriated for their "historical individuality," requiring particular forms of observation for their regulation. Epidemics affecting collective populations require a "multiple gaze," diffuse and detailed, but always adopting an implied coherence.[11] By scrutinizing those texts that claim to document the early AIDS crisis for contemporary audiences, this oblique cohesion and its structuring absences illustrate how policies prejudiced against queer citizens are sustained.

And the Band Played On (hereafter *Band*) and *Red Gold* are significant because they offer coherence to an otherwise fragmented narrative. They give heightened voice to a medicinal prudence that was a mere whisper during the initial crisis. There are virtually no articles in popular newspapers and magazines that document the early years of the blood ban. While meetings such as the one discussed at the start of this chapter received some attention, only one newspaper, the *Philadelphia Inquirer,* covered those proceedings.[12] More often than not, the issue of queer blood donation surfaces in cultural texts such as *Band* and *Red Gold* which appear to be informed by scientific foundations and objective knowledge. Accounts of the blood crisis are usually recounted in the form of documentaries or docudramas, using interviews with scientists and medical doctors who had firsthand experience with the escalating epidemic. In this manner, there is a careful construction of exigency with an understanding of AIDS produced through the perspectives of institutional actors who function as historical witnesses to this traumatic cultural phenomenon. While scant references to the blood ban are found in popular culture, features such as *Band* and *Red Gold* are explicit in their memorializing representations.[13]

Band was originally published in 1988, offering an almost quotidian account of the AIDS crisis as it unfolded. Well received by the press and reading audiences, Shilts's book was nominated for a National Book Critics Circle Award for detailing the institutional failure to stop the initial spread of HIV. The book was later modified for the small screen, becoming a highly regarded made-for-television movie on HBO starring Matthew Modine and Alan Alda. Even though the film initially aired as a cable production, it is still recognized as one of the first films that attempted to come to terms with AIDS for popular audiences.[14] The AIDS scholar Douglas Crimp once contended the film was one of the most common sources of information about AIDS among his undergraduate students in the years following its release.[15]

Despite being embraced by numerous audiences, both the book and the movie have been attacked by critics for the manner in which the pandemic and gay men are portrayed. Not only do the texts (both the book and the film) reinforce the unfounded claim that AIDS originated in Africa, they also depict gay men as equally responsible as the government for the epidemic.[16] This occurs in part because Shilts's narrative necessitated a dramatic story line more than a deep understanding of complicated scientific data. His account required heroes and villains, the honorable and the despicable, the knowledgeable and negligent. Viewers are encouraged to identify with scientists such as Don Francis, who always seems aware of the syndrome's progression, despite the CDC's lack of empirical data or government support in the film. To contrast this solid, scientific understanding, audiences are offered dangerously unaware gay men such as Gaetan Dugas, or "Patient Zero," a promiscuous flight attendant who Shilts positions as one of the most prolific spreaders of AIDS. In the end, he constructs little more than a text rife with homophobic images and disputable facts. For example, Shilts never addressed accounts that speculated that many of the men Dugas had sex with may have contracted HIV prior to meeting him. Additionally, Shilts defended rumors that Dugas had mocked sexual partners, telling them that they were going to die from HIV infection after he slept with them.[17] While representing queers as largely irresponsible, Shilts continually neglected to mention that most of the accomplishments in early AIDS activism were attained in large part because of a vibrant and vocal gay community.[18]

The 2002 PBS miniseries *Red Gold: The Epic Story of Blood* is an extended four-hour documentary on the history of blood, covering subjects that range from early understandings of transfusion science to new technologies in a "post-AIDS" world. The third installment of the series is especially pertinent as it detailed the crisis associated with the blood donation process and those affected by it. Oscillating between individual stories and the testimony of scientists such as Don Francis, the production established the importance of the blood ban, literally featuring it as part of an "epic" story. Although not as widely consumed as *Band, Red Gold* presents an opportunity for exploring a

text that reifies a particular cultural narrative. It is a production built on scientific testimony, historical data, and institutional voices.

Several noteworthy parallels connect *Band* and *Red Gold*. Both of the
films are based on books written by journalists who covered science, each of
which is of substantial length (Shilts's text being just over six hundred pages,
Starr's just over four hundred). The films were both developed for a television audience, one being made for HBO, the other for PBS. More important, each follows a similar narrative when detailing the history of the blood
ban, often using the same figures, meetings, direct quotes, and timetables.
The tie to journalistic form is especially important, as they, like science, are
positioned as more objective than other narrative accounts. They operate in
a manner similar to Simon Watney's explanation of AIDS scandals in the
popular press, positioning viewers as "normal" citizens who can disavow their
homophobic and racist tendencies as they consume dramatic accounts of infection and loss.[19]

The fact that these discourses appeared on television is also a significant part
of the entextualization process for this cultural narrative. Just as blood donation is an especially intimate form of civic participation, television is among
the most intimate forms of media. As a medium, television penetrates the
home, allowing people to watch programs anonymously, with differing economic commitments and social investments than when they are in theaters.
Television also supports the nature of scientific understanding in ways that
films traditionally do not. By their very necessity, popular films are created
with profit central to the motives of the creators.[20] While docudramas and
television documentaries necessitate monetary funding and an audience, their
content purports to show things "as they are," through the direct observation
of the camera. The rise of reality television highlights the popularity of such
forms, which have not been as successful in theatrical release. *Band* and *Red
Gold* are steeped in realism, melding narratives forged in the cultural imaginary into natural reflections of everyday life.

Crucially, productions such as *Band* and *Red Gold* are especially powerful
because they tend to confound scientific knowledge with prudential thinking. Robert Hariman has rightly suggested that the concept of prudence is
used for the purposes of "identifying and getting inside of that new class of
political problems that currently elude solution because of both their complexity and their lack of alignment with established political interests."[21]
Rather than complicate confusing data, moral action, and social prejudice, the
media programs under analysis here offer clear conclusions and inspire a kind
of commonsense thinking that frequently excludes men who have sex with

other men. This common sense is rarely foregrounded, usually surfacing as a result of miscalculated action or victimized heterosexual actors.[22] This subtle form of prudence is usually delivered in small doses, ensuring that citizens digest the substance of the message, rather than choke on suspect implications.

The power exhibited by televised forms is telling when one contemplates their ability to reinforce traditional norms of prudential thought. Television is often regarded as "low culture" because it is populist and readily available, and it rarely challenges aesthetic boundaries as other forms of art and media might. It is for this reason that John Nelson has posited that the most engaging theories of prudence are currently transpiring outside of the academy, in popular culture and politics. He suggests that as "modern turns to science and ideology have worked, respectively, to denigrate rhetoric and eclipse republicanism, cultural and intellectual support has eroded for prudence."[23] In short, the invocation of scientific discourses can radically reposition communal notions of common sense. As such, it is necessary to discern how science is insinuated into prudential narratives, often using popular culture as a vehicle. After all, people rarely inquire about the origins and intentions of messages encountered in the mass media.[24]

The narratives developed in these docudramas offer specific details about the development of events and particulars about people involved with the unfolding action. These texts situate audiences to remember critical events through the lens of heterosexual hegemony.[25] This hegemonic frame is strengthened by the fact that expressions of cultural memory are almost always preoccupied with concerns grounded in the present, even if they are grappling with issues positioned in the past.[26] In this sense, memory generally speaks through structures of power to those engaged in the cultural politics of the present. Institutions often attempt to facilitate identification in cultural memory by incorporating the values of "ordinary people" into the fabric of discursive structures.

The role and placement of bodies plays an especially important part in the establishment of prudential narratives. Bodies are continually positioned to reinforce, reform, and reinvent understandings of common sense in a polity. This cultural situatedness operates fluidly, and often unconsciously, as bodies perform specific public repertory effects, some of which will make it into the archive, but many of which will not.[27] For example, Christine Oravec has illustrated how the process of feminization as it developed through nineteenth-century rhetoric was discretely linked to the transformation of propriety as something closely related to prudence and norms of social demeanor. She explains that "much of what pertains to our concept of propriety, with all of its intricate connotations of exactitude, inhibition, and fear of social chaos, belongs also to our conception of women."[28] Women were simultaneously positioned as keepers of decorous boundaries and silenced by these same norms. As women became more politically active, they were further represented as decorous representations that confirmed the legitimacy of the political process. They were, in many respects, queer bodies goaded by normative discourses.

Gay men come to occupy a similar position in the cultural management of blood in relation to the scientific world. At all times in the narrative of cultural memory, gays are clearly positioned as people who had a role in the decision-making process, but who ultimately disturbed the rational calculation of the deliberative process. Their public emotionality seemed to infect the public sphere, tainting the logical episteme of science with a chaos as digressive as their sexual longings. Oravec notes that "the rationality, order, decorum, and attention to process characteristic of the bourgeois political order were arrayed against the impending absurdity, passion, disorder, and risibility of the female mind."[29] Gay men are situated in comparable ways, always having access to knowledge that could have saved lives, but never embracing it. The prudence of the scientific process is subverted by the irrationality of queer pleasure. Medicinal prudence, as we shall see, is superseded by social denial.

In accounts of AIDS memory, there is rarely one villain wholly responsible for the contamination of the blood banks. Traditionally, there are usually negative representations of the blood banks, the government, science, and the gay community. With such an array of "villains," incorporating appropriate heroes that audiences can identify with is an important element of the healing process. By constructing appropriate hero figures, the public is reassured that preventative measures have been developed because specific individuals have already suffered and sacrificed for the polity. However, if it is true that "cultural memory in the context of AIDS is not about achieving closure but about keeping any sense of closure at bay," there must be a continual negotiation between the reiteration of the blood supply's fragility and the assurance that people are safe when receiving blood transfusions.[30] As such, several figures have emerged as reminders that the blood supply is tenuous, necessitating continual guarding of its borders and those permitted to donate.

The dichotomy that has been wedged between the gay man who has contracted AIDS because of sexual excess and the innocent victims that suffer through no fault of their own is so well documented it barely requires citation.[31] In terms of blood donation, however, this traditional dyad is carefully mediated alongside cultural representations of the known and unknown. Nongay people who have contracted HIV/AIDS are not simply innocent in each of these texts, but are archived as individuals who had an insightful

understanding of disease prior to infection. Such images present a number of
discursively constructed dichotomies that are contradictory, but ultimately
these ruptures are reworked to villainize queer citizens. These fantastic images
create an understanding of gay men that omits prudence from their civic identities. In accounts such as *Band* and *Red Gold,* audience members are offered a
historical perspective that positions gay men as simultaneously the most ignorant of their own bodies and the most hostile of people involved in the AIDS
crisis. In the later part of 1986, for example, a public health official ordered that
an HIV-positive man be placed under twenty-four-hour surveillance after he
allegedly defied an order to refrain from sexual activity. If caught engaging
in sexual activity, the man could have been sent to jail and been psychologi-
cally evaluated.[32] Importantly, as blood donors, gay people are almost never
offered a face, always being positioned as anonymous figures (the shadow of
John Doe explored in chapter 2) or mobs that negate the discourses of science
and the law.

Nelson reminds us that "prudential attention to figure connects narratives and tropes."[33] Popular accounts of gay blood donation are continually
mediated through the stories and images of heterosexuals who have contracted HIV from blood transfusions. The remainder of this analysis explores
the similarities and differences embodied by heterosexual figures connected
to the blood ban and how they are tropologically linked to understandings of
queer donors. For the sake of space, this analysis focuses on two primary figures. The first is that of Susie Quintana, the heroic mother-figure who is rhetorically tied to the trope of the unknowing gay donor. The second is the image of the hemophiliac, the person most in need of blood products, but who
is also at the greatest risk for contracting AIDS from tainted fluids. Hemophiliacs are continually positioned as victims, placed in strict opposition to a
vocal gay lobby. These "pure" rhetorical figures provide the tropological foundation for constructing medicinal prudence and the contrasting social denial
embodied by queer citizens in the social imaginary.

THE CASE OF SUSIE QUINTANA

People who represent historical events often secure such positions because
their stories appeal to abstract ideals that are embraced by the public. One
figure that continually surfaces in accounts documenting the dawning of the
AIDS crisis is Susie Quintana, a forty-five-year-old Colorado resident who
contracted HIV from a blood transfusion. The mother of two was hospitalized in late May 1983 when her .22-caliber hunting rifle accidentally dis-
charged, wounding her in the side. Prior to receiving the transfusion, her son

asked doctors if the family could contribute blood for the procedure, rather than rely on anonymous donors who might harbor infections. The medical staff assured him that the process was secure, telling him that there were "no gays or homosexuals in the county."[34] This improbable statement, locating gay people outside the boundaries of the county, is perhaps most troubling because it is clearly impossible to substantiate in this impromptu situation. Despite the likely presence of queer bodies in the area, their proximity was a moot point. The assertion had the effect of illustrating how little the hospital workers knew about the process of collecting donated blood or of the industry as a whole. The blood employed by the hospital was not amassed from members of the community, but purchased from the Arizona-based United Blood Services (UBS), which had not yet begun declining donors because of sexual behavior.

It should be noted in advance that this analysis is not meant in any way to discount the pain and agony that Quintana and her family suffered. Her story is tragic, and the false information offered to her family continues to be an important account of how little medical agencies knew about the syndrome, the blood-collecting process, and the presence of queer citizens. Quintana, like countless others, deserved better. But attempting to gauge why *this* story continues to be an important element of AIDS memory is a significant question with political import. Quintana's story is memorialized in the PBS documentary and in Starr's book because it is simultaneously tragic and uplifting. It dramatizes American values and sustains notions of radical individualism. While her demise is explicitly utilized as a condemnation of the lack of knowledge about the presence of gays and lesbians, the manner in which queer men are represented poses important analytical quandaries. The role of the gay man who donated this blood offers an extreme contrast with the purity and advanced knowledge by Quintana and her family. Although cultural institutions are understood as being disciplined by Quintana's courage, the story concurrently positions gay men in a particular light, one that continues to haunt their ability to act as full citizen participants. In the narrative surrounding Quintana, there is a subtle, but significant redemption of medicine and science at the expense of gay men.

In the PBS documentary there is a clear discrepancy between the pure mother figure who is infected with disease and the gay population. In the scenes prior to introducing Quintana's story, the series outlines the fast-spreading virus among gay men. This is accomplished not only through voice-overs, but through metaphorical visual representations as well. So, for example, as the program transitions from the narrative concerning gay men in the early 1980s to the segment about Quintana, there is a long shot of a winding city freeway at night with traffic traveling in both directions. As the fade sets in, the camera blurs the scene and the display is that of fuzzy red and white lights streaming across the screen. The lights, which pick up speed with the blur, are clearly meant to mimic red and white blood cells traveling at an accelerated pace.[35] The scene fades out and the audience is transported out of the city to a rural area, the streaming urban lights literally becoming a river. The program exhibits a number of images from the beautiful Colorado countryside, eventually ending on an image of a woman painting a white picket fence. The documentary has transitioned from the cities where gay communities are often thought to reside to a place in mid-America where "ordinary people" live. The small town being featured could represent any number of the communities that would eventually have to come to terms with the ravages of AIDS.

In many regards, Quintana represents the ideals of American identity, continually being depicted in relation to her family and exemplifying cultural values. Following the traditional style of narratives that represent innocent victims of AIDS, Quintana's personality is captured by Starr in a holistic fashion. He writes: "Hers was a bucolic existence, built around her husband, children, grandchildren, and community. Everyone in town knew Susie, and liked her. She had grown up in Dolores, met her husband at a dance, and gained some renown with her prize-winning crocheting. She was admired for her levelheadedness and cheerful personality."[36] Quintana was family oriented, community focused, and generally well liked. She is an easy figure to identify with, as she seemingly exemplifies the values of small-town America during the mid-1980s. Additionally, the characteristics offered in this account make her an appealing figure because she simultaneously embodies feminine and masculine traits. Not only is she good at crocheting, but (consistent with country life) she also hunts.

Quintana's story is a powerful account of the cruelty that people with AIDS confronted at the start of the epidemic. To highlight this tragedy, audience members are given access to intimate moments in her struggle against illness. The narrative details her accident, her son's confrontation with the doctor prior to the transfusion, and the time she discovers the illness ("about two weeks before Christmas"). Most painful of all is the recounting of the moment when she discloses to her husband that she has tested positive. Using his nickname, she is said to have told him, "Short, they've given me AIDS."[37] The community where she had lived throughout her life isolated her. People in Dolores no longer associated with her for fear they might contract AIDS. Quintana and her husband no longer touched, used separate bathrooms, and slept in different beds. At one point in her struggle, social workers found this once-vibrant woman alone and emaciated in the dark. Her son explains that, she "quit kissing her grandkids, she quit kissing us bye. . . . It just seemed like from the day that she found out what she had we lost our mother."[38]

Quintana sued UBS in 1988, ultimately losing the suit when the jury concluded that the organization had met existing industry standards when it collected the blood. At this trial, the gay blood donor who had passed HIV onto Quintana testified anonymously, by answering attorney questions and sending them into the court. Although UBS had requested that "homosexually active males with numerous contacts" not give blood, the phrase "numerous contacts" presented dangerous assumptions about the nature of HIV transmission and promiscuity. The gay donor testified that the questionnaire was unclear, asserting that the phrase "numerous contacts" did not apply to him. In the donor's words, "I did not know at the time that I donated blood that I could be infected with AIDS without manifesting symptoms. I don't think anyone did." The man believed that such infections were likely only among "Haitians, intravenous drug users, and homosexuals with over 1,000 different sexual partners." He added that the "information provided at the blood drive did not change or add to my knowledge of the disease."[39] By all accounts, the man "gave blood with a clear conscience and the best of intentions. He had no way of knowing that he might be carrying AIDS."[40]

This lack of knowledge exhibited by the donor is an important but often-overlooked element of the rhetoric of the blood ban. This oversight is especially significant when contrasted to the enlightenment appropriated to Quintana. One of the most disheartening elements of Quintana's story is that she and her family *knew* about AIDS and the risk of blood transfusions, in ways that the medical community and the gay man did not. Prior to her accident, Starr explains that like "millions of families throughout America, the Quintanas had heard news of the AIDS epidemic, and discussed it around the dinner table. They had all agreed that, if any of them ever needed blood, the others would provide it. Ron and his father had the same blood type as Susie."[41] This particular story is ultimately tragic because infection could have been prevented, if only the medical doctors in that community had listened to the Quintana family.

Four years later, Quintana went back to court, challenging not simply UBS, but the blood industry as a whole. Her attorneys argued that the industry ignored the measures suggested at "that horrible meeting" in January 1983 and brought in a powerful witness to attest to the ignorance of the blood banking community—Don Francis, the hero figure in *Band*. Francis testified that the blood industry as a whole had ignored the recommendations offered at the January 1983 meeting, refusing to believe that HIV had penetrated the blood supply because they had wanted to keep costs low.

In almost every account of the 1983 meeting in Atlanta, Francis is cited as a lone wolf against the blood industry, pounding his fist on the table and demanding, "How many people have to die? How many deaths do you need? Give us the threshold of death that you need in order to believe that this is happening, and we'll meet at that time and we can start doing something."[42] The former CDC doctor's testimony debilitated the industry's lawyers, who were overmatched by the presence of Quintana, her visibly fading health, and the damning testimony of a doctor who had fought hard against AIDS since its inception. In the concluding days of her trial, Quintana fell desperately ill and had to again be hospitalized. While the jury was deliberating, Quintana slipped into a coma and passed away. The judge presiding over the case sequestered the jury, who granted Quintana $8.1 million posthumously the following day.

It is worth repeating that the pain and anguish that Quintana experienced is something that no person deserves. The ignorance of her doctors for suggesting that no "gays or homosexuals" lived in her county and the reluctance of the blood industry to be more explicit with the information they may have had regarding HIV transmission and the stereotypes they propagated remain deplorable. But even years after the epidemic began, many health officials continued to perpetuate the myth that people who did not live in big cities did not need to worry about HIV from blood transfusions. One doctor told *Newsweek* magazine in 1987 that "if you're from Iowa and you've had a transfusion, I just wouldn't worry about it."[43] This line of thought overlooked the economic and social structures of blood donations and the dependence that some smaller communities have on blood from remote locations.

But what does this story speak to in the larger cultural memory of queer blood donors? Proponents of the blood ban continue to highlight a common element of the narrative—the degree to which the nameless gay man knew nothing of his affliction. Indeed, the disparity of knowledge between the gay man and the Quintana family is striking. The Quintanas had access to basic knowledge presented by a scientist at the Center for Disease Control in those early years in AIDS history. They are positioned by Starr as embodying the common sense that science had bestowed upon the country in the very early days of AIDS when he says, "Like millions of families throughout America," they had heard of AIDS and "discussed it around the dinner table."[44] Not only is the quantity (millions) significant, so are the qualitative normative features of the Quintanas, who are framed by the terms "families," "discussion," and "dinner table."

While the institutions of medicine and science are castigated in these narratives, there is a subtle recuperation of their credibility with figures such as Susie Quintana. In these accounts, audiences are faced with a scenario in which government scientists understood what was happening at the time, as evidenced by the knowledge possessed by "ordinary people" such as the Quintana family. When Susie Quintana is remembered, the path that should have been taken by industry officials is remembered. There is little focus on government inaction or policies that could have been *imposed* on the blood banking industry.

The degree to which scientists fully understood the implications of AIDS is consistently reinforced by the testimony offered by Francis. He asserted, "That's one of the saddest things about the blood banks: that not only did we (the CDC) present the data to them, but we really laid it on a silver platter what to do about it."[45] This statement speaks to the fact that imposing donor deferral measures would have been an easy and cost-effective method of preventing additional infections. Even if blood products businesses could not yet implement tests that would have detected HIV, donor deferral policies could have successfully curbed the increased rates of HIV infection. All of the information was right there, noticed by members of the American public, but neglected by officials in the blood industry.

Quintana's story has been remembered in large part because she took on the blood industry and won a large sum of money. Her story meshes well with cultural conceptions of the lone individual fighting the industry, just as Francis had done a decade earlier. But the attention offered to Quintana is in many respects rare. Women afflicted with HIV and AIDS are discussed far less than men in all institutional discourses. Historically, women have had to be exceptionally vocal about the degree to which they are affected by such medical problems in order to receive proper care. AIDS definitions often ignored symptoms exhibited by women, in large part because studies that detailed the relationship between the symptoms and syndrome had simply not been conducted. Those studies that did exist usually took place in locations where rates of infection among women were low.[46]

In contrast to the intimate details offered about Quintana, audiences never learn much about the anonymous gay man who donated the blood, who like many others remained a "John Doe" for purposes that are likely connected to privacy and safety. The fact that he was a teacher and gave blood in a room at a school offers the strong possibility that he may have taught at the location where the donation was made. That fact aside, we know only that he was *not* what some might call a "fast-track" gay man, was civically oriented, and that he had honorable intentions. Despite this, he was nonetheless HIV-positive and had managed to pass on his aliment.

This portion of public memory seems especially important for a number of reasons. Considering the blood industry lost this case, it has a vested interest in keeping men who have sex with other men out of the system. General ignorance about one's HIV status becomes ample justification for constructing policies that purposefully exclude an entire class of people with little regard for their individual sexual practices or self-awareness. In one of the most important legal decisions of all time concerning blood, we are faced with a stock example, one which suggests that if it can happen once, it can happen again. The family knew right away that they should have donated blood. The gay man, conversely, apparently knew nothing about AIDS, his own HIV status, or its methods of transmission. What remains troubling is that there is never a sense of how representative this case might be, that in May 1983 a family in rural Colorado possessed this information, but that a gay teacher, one who passes on knowledge to others, seemingly had no clue that he might be at risk.

While this singular account by no means highlights the point of origin of the figure of the unaware queer donor, this particular case reinforces a popular trope in public health rhetorics. The appearance of the unaware donor is so transfixed in medical discourse that its mediations here are not surprising. To be certain, I am not suggesting that the account of the gay donor not knowing his HIV status in the early 1980s is necessarily false. Rather, this rhetorical form is so familiar that historical contradiction is disregarded for the self-evident arrangement of common sense and medicinal prudence. It is difficult to deny that accounts such as the one detailed above are rampant in scientific discourses that emphasize the image of the unaware donor that invariably causes harm. For example, a 2002 study released by the CDC found that nearly 80 percent of all young American gay men carrying HIV didn't realize they were harboring the virus. According to the study, these men perceived themselves to be at low risk for infection, even if they had unprotected anal sex. The study prompted one newspaper to react with extraordinary hostility. The editors wrote: "We are into the third decade of an epidemic that has been the focus of the most intensive awareness campaign in the history of public health—an epidemic that has decimated the gay community—and gay men are apparently oblivious to it all . . . Not allowing gay men to give blood is discrimination, but a justifiable one: If gay men are ignorant of their HIV-status, and unable to judge whether they engage in risky practices, we are behaving responsibly to treat their blood as suspect."[47] The reaction to the study is hardly surprising, considering the ease with which science can group all gay men together and act as if they are universally ignorant of HIV and AIDS. But the report neglects to account for a number of significant variables because medicinal prudence supports their cause.

First, the editorial never specifies what is meant by "young" gay men. Traditionally, younger people are not among those populations most likely to give blood. Only 16 percent of all blood donors are between the ages of eighteen and twenty-four, with over 80 percent of donations coming from people over the age of twenty-four.[48] Additionally, the CDC study was never intended as a method for collecting information about potential blood donors. At no point did they inquire about attempts made by HIV-positive men to give blood. Further, the editors do not take into account the cultural and social factors that might inhibit men from disclosing elements of their personal lives. This is especially important because the study presented statistics about the number of minority populations that were supposedly infected with HIV. The report contended that 90 percent of newly infected black gay men and 70 percent of newly infected Latinos were unaware they had contracted HIV.[49] But some studies have speculated that minorities are less likely to give blood because they often feel marginalized in the communities where they live.[50] The data appropriated by the newspaper never takes into account the cultural and social factors that might inhibit men from giving.

Further, such studies are never contrasted with research that details the number of HIV-positive heterosexuals who are unaware that they carry the virus. They explain with great shock and awe the number of gay men who are unwittingly infecting the rest of the country, but never contemplate the degree to which at-risk heterosexuals who are entitled to donate may be doing the same. Rather than present such complicated questions, the newspapers simply disseminate the image of the unknowing gay man who is unsafe, not only to himself, but to the community as a whole.

Of course, the most problematic element of this editorial is the degree to which it conflates people who are HIV-positive with gay men who do not carry the virus. In doing so, the paper makes erroneous conclusions and passes them on to the public. The description above could lead one to believe that 80 percent of all gay men are HIV-positive, and all of them are donating blood. Without properly reflecting on the dangerous logic in this rhetoric, gay men become articulated with recklessness and disregard for others in the community. Such images are perpetuated time and again in cultural narratives that isolate men who have sex with men as unknowledgeable citizens who threaten to unravel the social fabric of the nation. In fact, some studies show that heterosexual men are much less likely to be tested for HIV than their queer counterparts.[51]

The anxiety in the editorial is reiterated in cultural narratives that connect the figure of the heterosexual victim to a specific trope of imagined queer identity. This construction of the gay man as an unknowing killer, however, is not the only image of the dangerous donor perpetuated by cultural discourses. Just as powerful is the depiction of gay men acting with maximum consciousness to harm the populous. In this next section, the image of the gay man as aggressor will be explored to more fully understand the relationship between these two rhetorical tropes.

HEMOPHILIAC VERSUS HOMOSEXUAL

While Susie Quintana's story is noteworthy for the ways in which it depicts gay men as lacking awareness of their own bodies, divergent cultural narratives have positioned gay men as a hostile threat to the nation. Urban legends have long featured the angry gay or bisexual man who preys on innocent people by inflicting unimaginable forms of vindication on unsuspecting victims. From ejaculating into tubs of Burger King mayonnaise to writing vengeful notes in lipstick on bathroom mirrors, gay men, especially those infected with HIV, have long been represented as uncontrollably hostile.

Early accounts of the AIDS crisis often position the gay community as an aggressive collective determined to secure their "rights," regardless of who dies in the process. As opposed to the figure of the unknowing individual gay man who donates blood and inevitably infects innocent people, cultural representations of the initial confusion surrounding AIDS frequently depict an unruly mob who kills indiscriminately to avoid being socially ostracized. Despite the fact that "ordinary people" had a solid understanding of the disease thanks to the dissemination of scientific information, members of the gay community are often remembered as ignoring institutional warnings at the expense of sexual pleasure and fear of stigmatization. This is especially true in *Band,* when the film depicts gay men in San Francisco as almost universally opposed to closing the bathhouses despite information presented by Francis and other figures of public import. They are featured as an irrational mob, acting with unfounded distrust of science and medicine. Gay men are portrayed as especially hostile when participating in public forums where important decisions are disrupted by seemingly unjustified identity politics.[52]

Notably, the image of the powerful gay lobby does not creep into just any account. Gay men are almost always pitted against other groups affected by AIDS—most notably hemophiliacs. Popularly understood as a disease that prevents blood from clotting, hemophilia is also a debilitating ailment that causes severe internal pain, requiring blood products that reduce suffering. In the late 1960s, blood transfusion technologies had provided new life for people afflicted by hemophilia with the development of Factor VIII, a glycoprotein that eases pain and clots readily.[53] Factor VIII revitalized the lives of hemophiliacs, affording them freedoms never before thought possible.

But all that changed with AIDS. By 1990 between eight and ten thousand men, about half of all hemophiliacs in the United States, were diagnosed with AIDS. Overall, about 90 percent of "severe hemophiliacs" were infected with either HIV or hepatitis. Even after knowledge about AIDS had been widely circulated, several doctors who specialized in hemophiliac medicine were hesitant to stop treatment for patients, as they had literally seen people "climb out of their wheelchairs."[54] Hemophiliacs and the organizations that represented them were left struggling with an appropriate response to the AIDS crisis, never quite knowing which members of the blood products industry could be trusted. While some in the blood industry, such as Alpha Therapeutic Corporation, had implemented donor deferral policies as early as 1982, other manufacturers did not because of economic greed.[55] Even though many hemophiliac organizations knew there were risks associated with blood products and pushed for donor exclusion measures to be passed, they also continued encouraging hemophiliacs to use clotting factors.[56]

As with Quintana, several individual hemophiliacs became publicly recognized figures. And, like Quintana, their livelihood was discounted in deplorable and abhorrent ways. The focus on young hemophiliac men was especially prominent, with high-profile cases such as Ryan White in Kokomo, Indiana, and three brothers in De Soto, Florida, attracting national attention. Similar to Quintana, these boys gained prominence in large part because of the public prejudice they confronted. Often this discrimination was fueled by the conflation of homosexuality and hemophilia. Describing the prejudice that White faced after being barred from his school, Dorothy Nelkin explained: "Ryan's photograph appeared in an Associated Press article in which he was identified as a 'homophiliac [sic] who had contacted AIDS through a blood transfusion.' This typographical error, conflating hemophilia and homosexuality, is a frequent malapropism that has even been heard in the context of our international meetings involving sophisticated physicians, academics, and administrators involved [in] AIDS policy. It is an amusing slip except in the context of the stigmatization of children who test positive for the HIV virus. For they are, inevitably, morally contaminated by their 'bad blood.'"[57] The rhetorical conflation of hemophilia and homosexuality is an odd misnomer. However, this blurring of terms has a long history for men afflicted with hemophilia. As David Kirp points out, many younger hemophiliacs prior to AIDS were frequently referred to as "hemo-homos" because they were often frail.[58] This social stigma ran so deep that it prevented gay organizations and hemophiliac groups from building more foundational alliances in the struggle against AIDS.[59]

While much of the mix-up surrounding the words "hemophiliac" and "homosexual" is due to phonetic errors, there is another simple reason why the two groups were frequently articulated: in the public imaginary both are often composed of men, especially in relation to AIDS. Hemophilia, in particular, is a condition that is almost exclusively limited to men.[60] Organizations representing LGBT people and hemophiliacs, however, have historically had divergent responses to the AIDS crisis. While gay men stressed a model of empowerment over conspiracy, hemophiliacs have focused almost exclusively on being victims of the system. While gay people often became involved with the medical understandings of the disease, hemophiliacs have focused less on the development of a vaccine and more on government reparations. Gay men were determined not to be thought of as "people dying of AIDS," but hemophiliacs adopted the label for political purposes.[61]

While the two groups have been habitually confused in many cultural settings, in the political arena, gay men and hemophiliacs are received in radically dissimilar fashions. In fact, gay men are often blamed as the reason so many hemophiliacs were infected with HIV. During the passage of the Ryan White Care Act in Congress, then Senator Jesse Helms explicitly stated that gay men were responsible for White's infection and ultimately his death. Indeed, often the most venomous opponents of gay rights have aligned themselves with hemophiliacs.[62] Sadly, hemophiliac organizations in the past frequently adopted a language that was explicitly homophobic in order to advance their goals. Such organizing was so successful that Congress passed the Ricky Ray Act, which promised approximately $100,000 to each hemophiliac (or surviving family member) infected with HIV from blood products, an offer that was never extended to people who contracted AIDS from transfusions, but who were not hemophiliacs.

Despite these political victories, hemophiliacs are rarely portrayed as "vocal," "powerful," or "advancing an agenda." Time and again, however, gay men are positioned as excessively powerful in their fight against donor deferral policies based on civil rights arguments. Reflecting on the January 1983 meeting, Louis Aledort, the director of the Medical and Scientific Advisory Board of the National Hemophilia Foundation, commented, "I disagree vehemently with the National Gay Task Force. They may want to protect their rights, but what about the hemophiliacs' right to life?"[63] Likewise, in *Band,* viewers are offered the image of the gay rights groups facing off with the parents of hemophiliacs.

Like Quintana, hemophiliacs were constituted as knowing victims in narrative accounts, often having access to the same kinds of information that government agencies possessed. However, critiques of hemophiliac and gay responses to the epidemic often discount the degree to which the gendering of these identities is of central import to larger social and cultural structures. Recounting the history of AIDS from the perspective of Corey Dubin, one of the first persons to benefit from blood products, Starr writes that the man, "was watching the evening news as he gave himself a Factor VIII injection. A hulking man with a Pancho Villa mustache and a savage intensity, Dubin had been infusing since he was a boy. . . . It had changed his life utterly, giving him the freedom he craved to hike the Muir Trail in the mountains of California and bushwhack through the jungles of Costa Rica. Now, as he infused another of the thousands of doses he had taken since childhood, he turned to his wife and said, 'Shit. I just *know* I'm shooting myself up with AIDS.' "[64] This prose is inevitably an accurate form of foreshadowing. Notably, there is little here about Dubin that would imply anything that is even remotely feminine. Not only is he a "hulking man," he is married, athletic, and a testament to man's technological capabilities to triumph over nature. This trope of masculinity being attained and then ultimately crushed is true in many of the high-visibility cases of hemophiliac men.[65] Cultural scholars remind us that the body is a cultural form that constitutes and fosters meaning. And in this conception of the body, being active is an important part of being a man.[66]

Of central import to this argument is the idea that hemophiliacs were not able to live "normal" lives.[67] Blood products provided them with the ability to live freely without the constraints of disabling pain and fear of bleeding to death. But the function of the word "normal" in this rhetoric is key to understanding contemporary aspects of medicinal prudence. In *Red Gold* the term "normal" never vanishes. The major example offered to illustrate just how marginalizing hemophilia can be is evident in the statistics surrounding marriage. One doctor explains that prior to the development of Factor VIII, hemophiliac men were fourteen times less likely to wed than "normal" men. Dubin remarks in the PBS series that "our people were just regular people, living their lives, working jobs, trying to provide healthcare for their children. . . . And the next thing you know, three generations get wiped out."

In 1993, after mounting pressure from hemophiliac groups demanding congressional hearings that would detail who was responsible for the large-scale infections of hemophiliacs from blood products, the Department of Health and Human Services (HHS) launched an extensive inquiry. The HHS secretary Donna Shalala appointed the National Institute of Medicine (IOM) to conduct an inquiry reviewing the progression of scientific discoveries in relation to the development of policy procedures that would aid in drafting subsequent measures to protect the blood supply.[68] The report that was eventually issued by the IOM was a clear condemnation of the institutions responsible for protecting the blood supply in the years that AIDS emerged. Public health scholars have noted that the largest contribution of the report was not its recommendations for the future, but its "'establishment' of a narrative of the events of blood and AIDS in the first years of the epidemic."[69] Commenting on the report, one writer noted that, "The value of this document is that unlike most of the reams of articles and books that have been written about AIDS, it is free of polemic and political rhetoric."[70] It would seem that the report was little more than "scientific fact."

Of course, the IOM report is political, compiled with understated and overt polemics, persuasive metaphors, and socially constructed images of disease. Perhaps most interesting is the extreme similarity that documents such as the one produced by the IOM share with popular cultural texts such as *Band*.[71] Notably, the medical account was released about seven years following the narrative set forth by Shilts. But like the Shilts text, there is a constant return to the idea of the angry and scorned gay man. He is a figure who eschews "normality," health, and civic responsibility. For example, in discussing the donor pools of the late 1970s and early 1980s, the IOM study explained that several gay men acted as donors to help develop a hepatitis B vaccine "to gain a [sic] social acceptance."[72] Not surprisingly, they never explain how gay men thought they were increasing their ratings in the polls by volunteering to produce vaccinations for incurable diseases. Nor is it ever considered that health officials may have used the allure of increased public acceptance to woo gay men into acting as donors for medical experiments.

Despite the need of queer people to argue for public acceptance, they seemingly exhibit extreme powers over the creation of public policy. The IOM writes that given "the scientific uncertainties and lack of representation by other consumer groups, the demands of the gay groups exerted considerable force in the debates regarding donor screening."[73] They continue, "gay groups, plasma fractionators and blood banks had more freedom to make their self-interested cases because the scientific information that would have clarified the nature of the calamity facing the United States was still in dispute."[74] The rhetoric is startling, as they assert that members of the gay community should have known what scientists and medical doctors apparently did not (at least not in this telling of the narrative). It seems self-evident enough that empirical medical evidence could have drastically altered the course of history. But they never hint that gay groups may not have acted in such a "self-interested" manner if this data had in fact been available.

Further, when health officials were contemplating the implementation of donor deferral measures, there was concern that gay men might donate precisely because they were denied the option. They write that "the blood banks perceived that the gay community might not cooperate if gay donors were rejected on the basis of sexual orientation, and furthermore, that they might donate on purpose or out of spite."[75] This discourse mirrors that of conspiracy theories on the right that fear gay men will strike back at the heterosexual community. Gay men have often been recast as AIDS-infested creatures capable of "blood terrorism" in far-right texts, such as *The Pink Swastika*, which warn of angry gay men ready to infect the blood supply if their demands are not met.[76]

Accounts of the blood ban continually situate the hostile gay lobby against the image of the hemophiliac. These rhetorical developments are troublesome not only because of the manner in which they are popularly remembered, but also because of the ways they are adopted by science with little self-reflection. The gay man, as has been illustrated here, is both wholly knowledgeable and vastly unaware. He is dangerous because he is in denial of the damage he is inflicting on innocent citizens. These images support the assertions constructed by scientists, never leaving room for a more thorough discussion about the subject matter.

CONFLICTING IMAGES OF EXCLUSION

John Nelson has argued that "studies of prudence cannot neglect the margins."[77] The development of the blood ban's short history is, in many regards, narrated by those occupying the margins. It is the story of gay men, of mothers who lose their children or their lives, of hemophiliacs who desire nothing more than to exist "normally." While seemingly dissimilar in their rhetorical development, these margins depend on one another to articulate particular understandings of civic participation, the role of science, and the ideal citizen. It is through the development of the docile hemophiliac that gay men materialize as hostile, and through the awareness of individual victims like Susie Quintana that gay men are constructed as oblivious. Scattered throughout this narrative are hints of a gendered citizenship, one that helps cement the medicinal prudence established throughout these texts.

As the rhetoric of the blood ban has evolved, competing understandings of gay blood-donor motives have oscillated. On one hand, gay men are represented as acting with maximum consciousness to infect the blood supply regardless of the information that they possess. On the other hand, these same men are perceived as oblivious to the perpetual crisis, donating without knowing the status of their health. Although seemingly contrasting discourses, each of these rhetorical developments allows a disregard for scientific logic and public health. Positioned in opposition to the secular scientific knowledge appropriated to figures such as Susie Quintana or Corey Dubin, gay men are located at the extremes of the hostile mob and the unenlightened individual citizen. This aggressive persona is consistent with a history of disparaging representations, as gay men have long been thought "to symbolize not only the confusion of sexes but also sexual excess—the violation of a delicate balance of passion."[78] The imprint of "passion" is significant, as it illustrates the degree to which gay men continually negate the logos of science central to the development of donor deferral policies. The images reiterated in these discourses stress the passions that drive the gay community, rarely focusing on the efforts set forth by queer activists since the dawning of the AIDS era.

People like Quintana and the hemophiliac men function rhetorically as figures that connect the memories of the early 1980s to fantastic tropes of queer donor identity that persist today. The heterosexual actors embody those citizens who strove to reach a degree of normality prevented by the stigma of AIDS. In the tragic cases of Susie Quintana and the hemophiliac men this normality is highlighted in the reproduction of traditional cultural values: they grew up in small towns, embraced matrimony, and centralized the importance of the family. However, recognizing that reproductive normativity governs "ideas about representation and inflect the negative values associated with the nonreproductive and the unrepresentable," it remains important to contemplate how these ideas precariously position queer citizens.[79]

Public memory of the early AIDS crisis produces images of queer men plaguing efforts to curtail AIDS. Caught between the stereotypes of an adverse gay community and careless individuals, there is an articulation of identity that counters understandings of an idealized prudential actor. As opposed to the citizen working to aid others in the community, there is a conception of the citizen who is in *denial,* one who is both wholly aware and refusing to acknowledge the "reality" of the transpiring events. They act not with maximum consciousness to gather information and make positive decisions that aid others in the polity, but to absorb data with the intent of ignoring it for undetermined reasons.

The materialization of these memories—the articulation of the citizen in denial—can be seen in a number of outlets that address public health. For example, in the article that castigated gay men for donating blood despite their infections, the editors commented: "It seems improbable that these men are simply ignorant. As sociologists have noted, gay men typically are more culturally aware than the rest of the population.... If we rule out ignorance, there is only one real alternative: mass denial. There has always been anecdotal talk among gays that reckless sexual behavior reflects a kind of death wish. Perhaps the recent findings support that."[80] Readers are presented not only with a cultural stereotype about the "over-educated" gay man, but with the dismissal of that knowledge. In *denial* one finds the antithesis of prudential action. There is no civic wisdom in denial, no glory to be found from closing our eyes to the disasters confronting our communities. In this account queer men not only seek death, but the editors would have us believe that queer men themselves are the witnesses to such death wishes, providing the public with anecdotes that have *always* been present.

If there is any doubt that representations of the early AIDS crisis haunted the logic of blood-ban policies in the decades that followed, one need only look to work being produced by public health scholars such as Sherry Glied. In a 1999 article Glied, the chair of the Department of Health Policy and Management at Columbia University, argued against lifting the ban. For reasons that remain unclear, Glied argued that gay men wish to donate for the sole interest of furthering their political goals. She asserted, "Once a gift is motivated by something other than pure altruism, whether cash or other benefits, there is less reason to believe that it will be in the best interest of the recipient."[81] Those "other benefits" are never completely delimited in the article, but could easily be labeled "civil rights" (if not "special rights") given the ways in which gay men are positioned in the essay. Using scientific studies to support her thesis, Glied argues that members of "high-risk" groups are unlikely to curtail donating blood without specific deferral policies. She explained that "knowledge of HIV risk factors was widespread among risk groups (particularly gay men) before 1984."[82] Despite the information that they possessed prior to that Orwellian date, Glied, consistent with the IOM report, insisted that they continued to give regardless of the harms brought upon others.

To clarify some of the erroneous fallacies in this text, it is important to tease out a number of astonishing assumptions woven into the fabric of Glied's prose. At the most basic level, Glied sees little concern for employing statistics that support how gay men felt about AIDS at the time the article was composed and not at a time when people, including most scientists, seriously underestimated the illness. Even though the article was published in 1999 she never uses statistics published after 1985. There is an irony in reading a scholarly piece about responsibility and obligations to community when concern for an entire group of people is wholly omitted from the work. Rather than concern herself with the difficulties of examining the changing nature of

how people identify as members of a "high-risk population," how information was originally disseminated, or the groups that were point-blank ignored,
she relied on irrelevant materials to discredit an entire class of people.

Further, it never struck Glied that members of stigmatized groups such
as gay men do in fact wish to donate for "purely altruistic" reasons. To my
knowledge, and those in the scientific community I have spoken with, there
has been no data collected on the number of "men who have sex with other
men" who have attempted to donate blood for genuinely beneficent reasons.
In fact, a large number of people (of all sexual orientations) seem to be unaware that such prohibitions even exist. At the time Glied was writing, the
ban had been imposed for at least fifteen years. New generations of queer men
were willing to donate—and not simply to make a political statement. Rather
than ponder the possibility that omitted populations wish to be included for
reasons concerning community and health, Glied explicitly positions gay men
as nothing more than a self-motivated demographic group.

Additionally, Glied never explores the possibility that such exclusions do
in fact stigmatize men who have sex with other men. She never discusses the
deep complexities of identity, of the very conflicted relationship that many
men have with the act of blood donation. Placing the complaints of gay men
in one paragraph and immediately following them with a conversation on the
dangers of impure motives does little more than reproduce the very stigma
(and logic) she purports to be addressing. Motives are a difficult grammar to
translate and a dangerous rhetoric to promote without an exhaustive account
of how people would respond to blood donation in a range of situations and
under a variety of constraints. Glied relies on the trope of social denial to support her specious claims. If "knowledge of HIV risk factors was widespread"
among queer men, readers (not to mention the countless medical personnel
trained in departments such as Glied's) are left with the impression that gay
people are hostile at best and insane at worst.

While constructions of gay men living in denial to the threats they pose
against the community offer insight into how the memory of the blood ban
functions, one final implication needs to be addressed. It is difficult to overlook the central role that gender plays in this history and the development of
this discourse. While women have often been neglected in scientific understandings of AIDS and HIV, figures such as Quintana are endowed with a vast
amount of knowledge and purpose.[83] As this analysis has illustrated, she is a
powerful presence because she represents traditional Western values bestowed
with scientific insight. She is a centralized maternal figure from small-town
America who rises up to fight not the medical officials who offered her false
information regarding the process of blood collection, but the blood-products

industry. She was supported by high-ranking members of the scientific community in a legal forum where greedy representatives were disciplined by a jury of their peers. As a woman, Quintana is appropriated the powers of scientific knowledge, being positioned as a figure that continues to fight against the unflinching and unsympathetic blood banks.

Along with Qunitana, audiences often encounter images of hemophiliac men, usually the only heterosexual men afflicted with AIDS in these discourses. They are literally the docile bodies, dependent on altruism in order to live their lives fully. As a group, however, they are not overtly constructed in a manner similar to gay men. They are appropriated sparse tropes of masculinity, being represented as bodies that are prevented from being fully active. This inability to sustain motion, the susceptibility to being penetrated by AIDS as gay men are, places them in a position that prohibits them from embodying a masculine identity as other "normal" men might. Certainly, the comparison to gay men (who are often depicted as weak and dying from AIDS) helps suture these articulations.

Rhetorically, it is the docile embodiment of both Quintana and the hemophiliac that allows science to be recuperated. Quintana and the hemophiliac men can temporarily adopt the characteristics of scientific reasoning to support institutional discourses, but never fully achieve the masculine persona that marks such institutional rhetorics. Their experience with illness offers them an unquestionable credibility when recounting stories of AIDS and the impact it had on American culture. But their individual narratives and cultural positioning as "underdogs" also makes them suitable contrasts to gay men, who have long been seen as plaguing science's ability to deal with the pandemic.

Indeed, pitting science against gay people is risky, as it places scientists in the precarious position of fighting against a population who was prey to their shortcomings. It is not surprising that the only other consistent representations of men in these narratives besides gay men and hemophiliacs are the self-assured scientists who are always constrained by budgets and bureaucracies, but who nonetheless hold the truth. In the narrative set forth by the IOM, scientists asserted that at that fateful January meeting the "CDC presented data they had collected on AIDS in hemophiliacs and transfused patients. They concluded that AIDS was transmitted by sexual contact and through blood."[84] Such information is only partially true and was never offered with such confidence or strong will. Government agencies did not speak with one voice, did not have the backing of those in the hierarchy, and failed to implement important procedures concerning blood-donor deferral policies. In their critique of the government's inaction, for example, the Institute of Medicine argued that "when confronted with a range of options for using donor screening and deferral to reduce the probability of spreading HIV through the blood supply, blood bank officials *and* federal authorities consistently chose the least aggressive option that was justifiable."[85]

In this way, gay men are remembered in a manner that runs parallel to the state and the blood industry. Rather than being understood as a separate entity working to heighten awareness of AIDS, the gay community is more often represented as being an integral part of the system, one that was included in a rational, deliberative setting, but which ultimately subverted the interests of the nation. In the cultural memory of the blood supply, gay men carry as much responsibility for the early blood supply crisis as any state agency. Just as scientists were implementing their "prudent" decision, gay people seemingly stood in opposition to the commonsense adoption of deferral policies. It is this figure that is not equipped with knowledge that is constructed as deleterious, as wholly in denial of the crisis that continues to be perpetuated. Coupled with figures such as Quintana and the hemophiliac man, science can speak through their bodies, being not a part of that system, but operating in a secular manner endowed with knowledge only after people have been infected.

More significant still is the power appropriated to state agencies when confronted with discourses of disease. Such complicated rhetoric makes questioning suspect policies that have been developed by the FDA and other blood banking entities a violation of prudential reasoning, a way of literally putting people in harm's way. In the next chapter, I will explore how this trope of the citizen in denial is managed by scientists in deliberative settings. By examining the rhetoric of officials that implement donor exclusion policies, this analysis can more thoroughly explore how queer men are castigated as citizens in the polity.

4
Diseased Citizenship and the Rhetoric of Scientific Deliberation

The home page of the American Red Cross Northern California Blood Services Region answers basic questions for potential patrons concerning blood donation and its rewards. The site explains that blood donation is a "convenient way to do volunteer work in the community" and "celebrate your good health with others." Included on the site are forty-three of the most frequently asked questions by prospective donors such as "Is all blood tested?" ("yes") and "How long does it take to get test results?" ("about 17 to 24 hours"). Each of these inquiries is answered directly by the organization, with the exception of query number seventeen, which asks: "Why are gay men not permitted to donate blood?"[1]

Rather than offer a rejoinder, the American Red Cross reprints an exchange published in the April 11, 1996, edition of the *New England Journal of Medicine* between San Francisco reader Ben Carlson and a group of doctors representing the Center for Disease Control and the Food and Drug Administration, the government agencies that regulate the ban.[2] Carlson criticizes the prohibition, asserting it is discriminatory and eliminates scores of healthy donors who might save lives. The doctors refute his arguments, claiming that excluding those who engage in activities that are "unquestionably associated with risk" is a matter of safety, not bigotry. The ARC allows science to speak on its behalf, offering no commentary on the exchange.

Rhetorically, the decision to employ this increasingly dated dialogue without explanation is intriguing, albeit ethically suspect. Although printed in the *New England Journal of Medicine,* Carlson's name is withheld on the home page, relegating him to the realm of anonymous self-interest. The doctors, on the other hand, have their credibility substantiated on the site with the publication of their titles, names, and addresses. While Carlson spoke directly of gay men, the doctors never once used the word "gay," utilizing the more medically sanitized "men who reported a history of male-male sexual conduct." Although the web site has been consistently updated with scientific data related to other matters, information used by the doctors, which at this writing is now thirteen years old, has remained unchanged on the site for public consumption. More remarkable still, the doctors wrote the "issue of donor exclusion raised by Mr. Carlson was not evaluated in our original report." Despite the absence of pertinent data in their study related to giving blood, the research is presented as self-evident proof against queer men acting as donors. Significantly, this scientific testimony is not addressed to just any lay audience, but specifically to the *Northern California Blood Services Region,* a politically progressive community with an active queer constituency. The implementation of scientific credibility and medical research to quell any potential outcry exhibits not simply the force of institutional ethos, it also illuminates the investment those institutions have on a girdled epistemology that circumscribes the discursive boundaries of health and illness.

Science is privileged frequently as an objective and apolitical institution resting beyond the reach of cultural bias. Because science and medicine allege to discover knowledge "that is not contaminated by the need to make human judgments," they are positioned to authoritatively speak on political issues with little worry of being regarded as partisan.[3] The absolute nature of scientific claims provides comfort and assurance for people by evoking "rational" arguments, empirical evidence, and results that can be methodologically replicated. So, it is not surprising that an editorial addressing the blood ban in one Florida newspaper echoed the common refrain that the "Food and Drug Administration should decide whether to ease the ban on blood donations from gay men strictly on the basis of *science* and *safety.*"[4] However, as Lawrence Prelli observes, even scientists make "claims that are empirically inaccurate, inconsistent, quantitatively imprecise, or lacking explanatory strength."[5] As such, it is important to examine how scientists employ language and authority to constitute audiences, ground findings, and structure modes of empirical proof.[6] Constructing particular lines of systemic inquiry enables what Troy Duster calls a "machinery of public policy" whereby science and bureaucracies invent internal logics to sustain discursive power.[7]

This chapter queers the scientific process of marking "men who have sex with other men" a danger to the national blood supply. Of particular interest is the FDA's Blood Products Advisory Committee, the panel that mandates federal recommendations regarding blood products and safety. Focusing specifically on "scientific" understandings of sexuality, the group dissociates key elements of cultural life that constitute civic identity, while giving presence to factors that serve their interests. They select finite aspects of the social world to construct disparaging and suspicious claims while deflecting observations that might alter otherwise erroneous suppositions. Forging a rhetorical schism between sexual practice and identity, the group locates the dangers of sexuality solely in sexual acts, not in the social performances and influences that precede or follow them. The BPAC centralizes the dangers inherent in sexuality and ignores an array of variables that would produce divergent conclusions about queer men and blood donation. Queer men materialize as *diseased citizens* who must be closely monitored and swiftly contained to ensure the safety of the blood supply.

Although ample consideration has been given to the critique of democratic practices that encourage multiple subject positions and a joining together of various identity politics, what continues to require attention is the institutional influence that encourages citizens to perceive themselves as divorced from one another in a polity. Like Iris Marion Young, I believe that "social structures often position people unequally in processes of power, resource allocation, or discursive hegemony," and this placement influences outcomes of justice and public recognition.[8] To further enhance these understandings of cultural identity, additional theoretical consideration must be given to the rhetorical fissures fabricated by agencies such as the FDA which situate groups as discreet entities with characteristics that can be scientifically measured and empirically discerned. Far from an innocuous discourse, such deliberations hinder the fight against AIDS by imagining queer subjects in denial of their dilapidated health, incapable of understanding their bodies or their roles in the polity. Tens of thousands of people who come into contact with blood-donor questionnaires each day are offered false assurance about the permeability of their own bodies with this troublesome conflation of disease, risk, and queer men.

It is well recorded that marginalized communities have never fully trusted the sanitized arm of science and its relationship to the state. Repeatedly, groups such as African Americans, gays and lesbians, and Jewish people have been constructed as less than human in scientific and medical rhetorics, being understood as impure, prone to sickness, and sexually imbalanced.[9] These qualities were inexorably tied to the "essential" identity of the people under scrutiny, ontologically secured by the fortitude of scientific scripture. In his account of the Tuskegee Medical Experiments, James Jones cites a doctor who contended, "The weakest members of the social body are always the ones to become contaminated."[10] Proclamations such as this are frightening not simply because of falsely perceived pollution, but because contamination always suggests purification. Gays and lesbians, for example, have habitually fallen prey to advocates of reparative therapy who wish to "fix" them.[11] Even today, much scientific research connected to sexuality is concentrated heavily on the discovery of the so-called gay gene, and some critics worry that such findings hold alarming opportunities for creating a human genome free of queer mitochondria.[12]

Scholarship on the rhetoric and politics of inquiry has illustrated the dangers associated with scientific discovery, especially as it relates to AIDS and its articulation with queer identities.[13] Science has frequently studied HIV/AIDS for economic profit, not altruism and the well-being of community.[14] A long-standing trope of AIDS history is the criticism that has been directed at government agencies for neglecting the plight of minorities and inhibiting the availability of drugs for low-income people. Activists such as Douglas Crimp have dedicated entire books to "the memory of the thousands who have died because of government inaction in the AIDS crisis, and to the survival of the millions who are fighting to stay alive."[15] Such contempt for the state and its institutional bureaucracies is a common expression of frustration and anger from AIDS activists ranging from ACT-UP to the Lesbian Avengers. Much of this censure has been directed at agencies focusing on scientific research such as the CDC, the FDA, and the National Institute of Health (NIH). The FDA, which houses the BPAC, has been especially prone to scrutiny and demonstration from interests as diverse as Queer Nation to the Committee of Ten Thousand, a hemophiliac lobbying group. Because the agency has a heavy hand in regulating everything from pharmaceuticals to blood products, it has often found itself at the center of high-profile controversies. Elinor Burkett notes that the FDA is notorious for bending to pressure and has never "had the freedom from politics essential to protecting the public health." The FDA, she explains, is the place where "politics and science collide in the tension between public good and corporate profit."[16] More often than not, the decisions made by the FDA have favored economic and conservative interests, working in many ways to the disadvantage of people living with HIV/AIDS.

In the last decade the fight against AIDS has taken a turn for the worse because of the right-leaning social politics of the Bush administration. Scientists at the NIH and the CDC were advised to omit key words from grant proposals to avoid offending high-ranking conservatives.[17] This list of inappropriate terms included "sex worker," "needle exchange," "anal sex," and most noteworthy for this study, "men who have sex with other men." One researcher at the University of California was advised to cleanse his application of words that were contentious for people in the administration, such as "gay," "homosexual," and "transgender."[18] These practices are especially problematic when one considers the strong role that reputation and rumors play in obtaining federal funding.[19] It is little wonder then that the BPAC has taken up the issue of queer blood donation so infrequently in the twenty-first century.

Cautioning against scientific deliberation is not intended to imply that science and its rigorous methods are universally invaluable. Strides in medicine and healthcare have provided countless people with longer, healthier lives. I personally benefit from blood technologies daily in my struggles with type-one diabetes. However, those who have quotidian experience with medicine and its close management of the body know that science and its multiple discourses are often incorrect in their attempts to regulate the complexities of everyday life. For all of its contributions, science, like any other institution, is composed of women and men who make errors and are guilty of faulty reasoning. Although one member of the BPAC implored his colleagues to "use common sense" and trust "the impressions of informed individuals," it is necessary to question *whose* common sense is being employed and *who* constitutes "informed individuals."[20] Contrary to a pronounced certainty or ability to rely on common sense as a trope of decision making, the BPAC deliberations highlight a pronounced anxiety about medical science and the populations being discussed. Their proceedings have much to say, both explicitly and implicitly, about queer men as they are understood through the lenses of disease and communal identity in medical rhetoric.

The remainder of this analysis concentrates on transcripts from the most recent BPAC policy-formulating meetings that addressed the issue of blood-donor deferrals for queer men. The committee was especially interested in the possibilities of altering the indefinite ban into a five-year or one-year deferral. The first meeting took place on December 11, 1997; the second September 14, 2000. This chapter also incorporates exchanges from a workshop on "behavior-based" donor deferrals the committee sponsored on March 8, 2006. Importantly, the 2006 session was not a policy-making forum. Technically, it was an information-sharing workshop that included doctors and scientists from all areas of the blood industry. However, when the FDA reiterated their decision to uphold the blood ban on May 23, 2007, they specifically cited the March 2006 meeting in their rationale.[21] The agency did not hold a public meeting before announcing the decision in 2007 as they had years before. The workshop featured several members of the BPAC (past and present) who grappled with the same diseases, projected the same deleterious metaphors, and clearly upheld the same logic engineered at the earlier meetings in 1997 and 2000.[22] Its inclusion here demonstrates the continued marginalization of queer men in scientific deliberation despite scientific advancements.

FRAMING, BLAMING, AND
THE LOCATION OF SEXUALITY

Deliberative forums are a flawed but necessary part of public culture.[23] Typically considered advantageous because they bring together people with inimitable expertise and divergent perspectives, deliberations are supposed to ensure that opposing opinions are aired, conflicting evidence debated, and self-interested parties monitored. In governing forums such as the BPAC, contributors scrutinize claims and arguments so conclusive judgments can be rendered and policies instituted. In its most ideal form, deliberators agonistically approach issues with the public good central to their mission. Participants "come to a political problem with an open mind about its solution; they are not bound by the authority of prior norms or requirements."[24] Those who partake in deliberations are idyllically free of coercion, social pressures, and privately guarded motives. Especially in scientific forums, members are most highly prized when they traverse a topic with tempered emotion and methodological precision.

Unfortunately, deliberations rarely achieve this idealized vision. Groups that share core values can unwittingly ignore imperative issues while giving presence to extraneous factors. Those in positions of power frequently control the placement of agenda items, the flow of conversation, and the content of discussions. In the case of the blood ban, the people most affected by a policy are commonly excluded from participation because they are deemed self-interested. Perhaps most important, those engaging in deliberations are always limited by the ways they symbolically construct meaning to make sense of the social world. These interpretive frames, what Kenneth Burke calls "terministic screens," prompt attitudes that predispose people to particular paths of action.[25] Even when cultural factors and emotions are supposedly bracketed, the language used to constitute issues in discourse both enables and constrains people's capacities for understanding. For example, although acting in the interest of the public good is laudable, it is impossible for participants to separate themselves from the frames that structure how notions of the "public good" are comprehended. When left unchecked, these interpretive frames can produce damaging normativities and irrevocable harms if the logic of a group is generalized as self-evidently beneficial to everyone and not as a set of rhetorical constructions unique to the group.

Too commonly, deliberations eclipse the voices of marginalized populations whose concerns are trivialized by experts and elites. In the LGBT community, some worry that science and medicine can "adopt a coercive, sometimes even brutalizing, attitude toward our lives, turning personal decisions into medical ones and thereby delivering our power to choose into the hands of professionals."[26] To combat the fetishization of rationality and fear of the other, some scholars have offered humanistic heuristics to reclaim the productive elements of deliberation. Robert L. Ivie, for instance, has advocated for a discursively focused "rhetorical deliberation." This conceptual lens promotes a "positive tension within a mixed constitution that holds elites more accountable to the people and treats the human divide as a condition for politics rather than as a basis" of terror.[27] Rhetorical deliberation invites modes of analysis that regard taken-for-granted logics in science and medicine as rhetorically devised, not inherently rational. It directs critics to unpack those features elevating discourses to the status of "truth" rather than accept such notions as naturally intuitive. Metaphors, analogies, tropes, and language itself is conceived as loaded with attitudinal forces that have material consequences.

Deciphering the vigor of scientific discourses using the spirit of rhetorical deliberation allows us to locate those iterations positioning queer men as diseased citizens and interrupt precarious interpellations. Queer sex is structured as perilous and achieves this inauspicious status through a continual stream of statistics and examples constituting MSM as impure. The notion that sexuality is an imminent threat to the blood supply is an incessant theme of the BPAC's discussions and serves as a master frame for these proceedings. The advisory board's conversations do not allow for complex consideration of sexual behavior and identity, continually implementing disturbing scientific information that situates queer blood as jeopardizing innocent lives. By concentrating their attention and efforts on sexual acts, scientists narrow their doctrine of queer identity to little more than a set of actions (if not a single act) that is void of context, culture, responsibility, and sexual awareness. Invoking a number of empirical studies and data sets, the committee couches sexuality in a language of contagion, hazard, and death.

Prior to discussing possible alterations to the deferral policies, the BPAC first contemplated hypothetical increases in pathogens that might result from assimilating queer blood. Although relaxing the rigid prohibitions against queer men could have produced a new pool of much-needed donors, the committee also believed it invited additional risks. At the initial meeting in 1997, the group noted it was required to approximate "how many infectious units could conceivably enter the blood supply."[28] The committee, which was composed of doctors, scientists, and (nonvoting) members of the blood industry, considered the following policy proposition: "Do the committee members believe that [the] FDA should modify its current recommendation that men who have had sex with men even one time since 1977 should not donate blood or blood components to be used for transfusion or further manufacturing?"[29] As the question indicated, a main concern for the committee was determining what course of action should be taken if the policy was amended. The BPAC had a variety of alternative deferment plans to consider. They pondered the possibility of deferring men who had had sex with other men over the past five years, the past year, or based solely on "risky" behaviors.

Regardless of the final decision, it was clearly indicated at the start of the meeting that the government would not tolerate any policy that promoted even a slight risk to the blood supply. This would seem reasonable enough if it did not imply there were no risks posed by other donor populations at the time. Dr. Andrew Dayton remarked that while the committee was sympathetic to charges of discrimination, "the country has made it clear through its representatives that any threat to the safety of the blood supply is intolerable, and it is incumbent upon us to protect, above all else, the health of recipient patients."[30] The doctor's comments are curious because they clearly delimit from the start of the proceedings a number of important assumptions that infect the progression of the deliberations. Notably, there was a clear distinction made between those discriminated against (queer men) and everybody else. "The country" here is not to be confused with those people who are identified as MSM. Instead, the nation is closely aligned with vulnerable "recipient patients." This suggested permeability was another way to implicate a threat without explicit mention of MSM. The presumption that the blood supply was safe, and not endangered by heterosexual donors, remained intact.

In each meeting, the committee addressed a variety of concerns about altering the deferral policies. These apprehensions ranged from the prejudicial nature of the MSM question to the risk of HIV exposure posed to blood center workers. In the initial gathering they also discussed the number of donors who might be harboring HIV early in its life cycle when it can exist without being detected by safety measures. Despite these worries, the board acknowledged that donors in the "window period" presented little danger because "it is generally felt that there are basically no seroconversions after a year," and most of the measures they were pondering would prohibit such infections.[31] In general, the doctors believed that scientific safety measures were effective and the assessments being made were, at best, guesses. As Dr. David Stroncek explained, "I think you have to really be cautious about these kinds of calculations. . . . It is my experience that there hasn't been a lot of HIV slipping through."[32] Stroncek, along with several others, trusted that scientific safeguards were effectively preventing harm.

In the earlier meetings, the BPAC took great strides to plot scientifically and statistically the risk posed to the blood supply if the ban were relaxed.

Each year about twelve million units of blood are donated to America's supply—with approximately ten units of HIV-positive blood passing undetected, causing two to three cases of infection. The odds of contracting HIV through a blood transfusion are roughly one in four million. Lifting the current ban could result, at most, in one to two additional cases of HIV a year. However, this is the *highest* number estimated and a strong possibility exists that no contaminated transmissions would result. At the preliminary meeting Dayton claimed that with a five-year exclusion policy an estimated 58,000 new donors would show up at blood centers to give. With a one-year exclusion policy this number would jump to about 112,000 people (in 2006 Dayton revised these numbers to 71,400 and 139,000, respectively). Unfortunately, these statistics are based on information that is difficult to corroborate.[33] In the end, the committee fell back on the conservative estimate that about twelve hundred units of infectious blood could make it to the testing stage. This statistic was reified despite committee agreements that they did not know what problems might be created by easing the ban. Dayton admitted that the scientists "don't know what the error rate is at this stage, but we worry about it. We assume that it's significant."[34] Repeatedly, the group is told they cannot be offered specific statistics about possibilities of infection because they "don't know the real error rate."[35]

The issues created by the window period had dissipated by 2006. With the implementation of Nucleic Acid Testing (NAT) in 1999, the window period shrank to under twelve days. Dr. Ronald Bayer explained that NAT testing had "all but closed the so-called window of undetectable infection."[36] There has been a virtual absence of infections in the blood supply. Dr. Michael Busch, who participated in the earlier BPAC meetings, told the 2006 workshop that the San Francisco blood centers only deal with one or two HIV-positive donations a year and those usually come from heterosexuals.[37] Since the implementation of the NAT screening "there have been four really proven HIV transfusion transmissions missed by mini-pool NAT."[38] Busch continued, "I just want to point out that none of these were MSM, or acknowledged MSM. Two of them were women with heterosexual infection and one was a male who, on follow-up extensive interview, denied MSM activity. So, what is getting through now is not related to MSM."[39] Nonetheless, the actual numbers of potential units that could infiltrate the system continued to worry doctors, even as their statistics were worlds apart. While Dayton predicted about three HIV-positive units per million would slip through with revisions to the policy, Dr. Celso Bianco of America's Blood Centers put the risk at about one in fifteen million.[40] The maintaining of the policy in 2007 suggests the FDA sided with Dayton, who sits on the BPAC.

Tellingly, the issues of increased pathogens and the window period both act as starting points of discussion that presume disease. Although contagions are certainly a naturally occurring reality, the ways queer men are articulated as embodiments of these vices is assuredly a product of human discourse. The eventual decision of the committee to maintain the ban required the use of rhetorics that reified harm and distanced questions about safe sex and the civic-mindedness of queer men. Three recurrent themes emerge from these transcripts: the group utilizes unnecessary metaphors of disease, implements suspicious data to frame queer men as dangerous, and employs a flawed scientific process to justify cultural prejudice.

DANGEROUS ARTICULATIONS OF DISEASE

The disputed information engaged by the BPAC did not prevent several participants from forging relentless images of queer men as diseased citizens. Members of the group divulged a number of reasons they were hesitant to modify the deferral policies. These grounds included everything from the donor's ability to recall the last time he had sex with another man to the fear that queer men were putting too much faith in scientific achievements.[41] Some also alleged that MSM often give blood for the "wrong" reasons. Dr. Lynda Doll, for instance, argued that 31 percent of the men in one study donated solely because they wanted to have their blood tested for HIV. In addition, over "60 percent indicated they had donated at a work site, and around 50 percent indicated that they felt pressured to donate by either fellow workers or the blood bank."[42] Another 38 percent said they had concerns about privacy when asked questions related to sexuality. Regardless of the data, none of these answers addressed what the committee wanted to hear—that all MSM were knowingly free from infections.

This exemplifies the first major problem exhibited by the scientific discourse deployed by the BPAC. Many members of the board were insistent on framing queer men as vessels of disease. The group rarely entertained the idea that there were health-conscious MSM who get tested, are safe in their sexual practices, or are aware of their HIV status. When queer men were discussed, they were immediately articulated with disease, and affliction was established *a priori* considerations of sexual behavior. During one question-and-answer period at the 1997 meeting, for example, Dayton admitted in his research presentation that he "did not take into account the [men] that had been tested and tested negative" for HIV. Rather, he took into account "the ones who had been tested positive and therefore self-excluded."[43] Similarly, Doll presented evidence from a study of donors who had reported having sex with another man after testing HIV-positive. Setting up a self-fulfilling prophecy, she explained that "48 percent reported unprotected receptive or inserted anal sex in the last year."[44] However, never once did the committee attempt to visit the fact that these statistics were emerging from studies that clearly identified disease first and sexual behavior second.

This logic, which considers people only after they are infected, allowed the committee to make presumptions about queer sex and the risks it posed to the blood supply without discussing the vast majority of MSM who live free of disease. The group never took into account those men who live in monogamous relationships, those who practice safe sex, and those who pay close attention to the state of their health. The BPAC's evidence equivocated sexuality and illness, presenting a distorted caricature of queer men as predisposed to disease and death. Not surprisingly, the correlation between MSM and AIDS surfaced repeatedly, with the doctors contemplating the number of individuals living with HIV and wildly spreading infection.

This is not to say that men, queer or otherwise, never have unsafe sex, grapple with infections, or ignore the historical lessons of AIDS. But various heterosexual communities are equally prone to the devastating effects of bloodborne infections and, as a result, are put at risk by this accusatory rhetoric. The citizenry is offered a false sense of security by encouraging those people who are not MSM to believe that both they and the blood supply are impenetrable. While organizations such as the Gay and Lesbian Medical Association implored that "like risks should be treated alike," several of the BPAC doctors were quick to defend the purity of heterosexual conduct, proclaiming "there may be a subtle misunderstanding that comparable behaviors always connote comparable risks."[45] One doctor argued that in the year 1997 "only half of the HIV-positive donors" were male, and "among those that are males, only 30 to 40 percent are the ones that reveal that they had risk behavior, sex with another male, in the past."[46] Not only was the conflation between "risk behavior" and same-sex intimacy explicit, but the committee ignored the flip side of this statistic, which found that 60 to 70 percent of the HIV-positive donors surveyed said they were not MSM. Studies that find gay men are more likely to be tested for HIV than their heterosexual counterparts were not included.[47]

The articulation between queer men and HIV/AIDS continued in 2006. While the workshop, which was larger and more occupationally diverse than the BPAC, was more likely to raise concerns about questionable assertions, the connection between queer men and their propensity to harbor HIV persisted. For example, Dr. Cees van der Poel, who was offering comparative information about disease rates in Europe, noted that "in France MSM is about

27 percent of the new HIV infections in 2003–2004, whereas only 4 percent of the general population has a history of MSM."[48] At other times the link was more subtle, but certainly implied. Van der Poel explained "from 1997–2004 there was an increase in unprotected anal intercourse by about 70 percent."[49] The enthymematic conclusion is that HIV rates will continue to rise among MSM.[50] This statistical data is compelling and most of us would agree that tracking HIV infections is a worthwhile and necessary endeavor. However, throughout these proceedings, little information was presented about how these rates are directly connected to men who would be blood donors. Glancing at these statistics, scientists are left with little data about these men, their propensity to be donors, if heterosexuals are getting tested less than queer men, if men in 2004 are more likely to admit anal sex than those in 1997, the HIV status of the men having unprotected anal sex, and if that intercourse is correlated to the statistics on AIDS. These questions are imperative because the reliance on empirical evidence generally works to the detriment of queer men. Dr. Steve Anderson, for instance, offered statistical data to demonstrate the increased risk of HIV slipping into the blood supply. Pointing to the limitations of the work, he commented that "we assume in the model that the prevalence for HIV is constant for all MSM populations."[51] This assumption, which Anderson admitted eliminated seventeen complex variables, presented the epistemological barricade marginalized citizens confronted.

Queer men, those abject citizens seemingly living and dying in the polity simultaneously, were a chronic threat in each of the conversations.[52] Thomas Yingling reminds readers that "American feeling for the body inscribes disease as foreign and allows AIDS to be read therefore as anti-American."[53] AIDS is marked as the breakdown of a complex system—in this case, that of national security.[54] Keeping in mind Dayton's proclamation that "the country" will not tolerate harms posed to the blood supply, it would seem that queer men in these discussions were enemy number one. But the overt assumption that gay men are introducing foreign agents into the blood supply is certainly not surprising. Scientists often utilize the metaphor of war when discussing the functions of the immune system, so the construction of an enemy is in many ways predictable.[55] Continually, the committee examined how the undisciplined bodies of MSM had the potential to foil science. They become carriers of undetermined diseases that can co-opt the nation through their lack of sexual virtue. One doctor professed to the fragile nature of the system against such unruly forces, asserting that "there are ways that the system gets—or bad things circumvent the tests and happen, or agents can circumvent the tests and get through to the blood supply."[56] His incomplete sentence certainly raises an eyebrow. "There are ways that the system gets . . . contaminated? . . . diseased? . . . penetrated?"

What remained elusive throughout the forums was the actual threat posed by queer donors. While HIV played a substantial role in the discussions, a menu of diseases was articulated with queer men. The implicit assumptions that gay men pose greater risks for contracting and transmitting diseases such as Hepatitis B (HBV), Hepatitis C (HCV), and the Human Herpes Virus–8 (HHV-8) were reoccurring themes. During a segment of the first meeting, Busch skirted the concern regarding HIV and argued that "hepatitis C is the problem here, because the prevalence of C in our donor pool is quite high compared to all the other viruses, and it is virtually 100 percent transmissible for C seropositives if they were to get through."[57] The connection to queer men, however, remained fleeting. Later during the same presentation Busch explained that "virtually all of the hepatitis C in gay men is in gay men who also use drugs."[58] Despite the clear link to substance abuse over sexuality, the issue of drug use was scarcely mentioned and the articulation with HCV stood. At the 2006 forum Dr. Ian Williams again pointed out that HCV is not easily spread through sexual contact, stressing that queer men who had fewer partners had reduced rates of infection. He reported that "when you look at men who have sex with men, they appear to really be at no higher risk than sexually active heterosexuals."[59]

In an almost conspiratorial fashion the impurity of the queer donor had the potential to enliven new and dangerous diseases. The scientists spent a considerable amount of time discussing HHV-8 at the meetings, which they described as a "new and emerging virus that is prevalent in the gay community."[60] While the committee agreed that HHV-8 is "unequivocally the causative agent of Kaposi's sarcoma" at the first meeting, many members of the BPAC, such as William Martone, a former senior executive director of the National Foundation for Infectious Diseases, were adamant in concluding that there was no risk of transmitting such diseases through blood transfusions.[61] The issue of HHV-8 became an extended part of the dialogue at the 2000 meeting. Many on the committee insisted that additional research on this virus be conducted, even though doctors had known about it since 1986. The topic of HHV-8 was persistently revisited, despite resistance from several participants who insisted there was no evidence proving the virus is transmitted via transfusion and "comes predominantly from individuals who are HIV-positive, not . . . people who have healthy immune systems."[62] Nonetheless, the association between disease and the queer citizen was more than a possibility in the forum, it was uniformly presumptive.

The affinity between queer men and HHV-8 was telling, not only in its portrayal of MSM, but of heterosexuals as well. As with the possibilities of HIV infection, there was again a purification of heterosexuality, which was continually reiterated as outside the grips of disease. The scientists asserted that HHV-8 is found predominately in the gay community, but "in women and donor donors, the rates are quite low, again."[63] "Donor donors" may as well read "heterosexual male donors," though "normal donors" and "healthy donors" were also repeatedly employed.[64] Potential queer donors, however, were completely excluded from such arguments because there was no sample from which conclusions could be drawn. Put simply, MSM were never offered an opportunity to be represented as similarly healthy.

The issue of HHV-8 again emerged during the 2006 workshop. Dr. Sheila Dollard of the CDC spoke about the contagion and warned there may be more potential to transfuse HHV-8 into bodies than previously believed. Pointing to Dollard's talk, Dr. Jay Epstein worried about the "significant prevalence of HHV-8 positivity in males who have sex with males" and the "convergence of evidence suggesting the likelihood of transfusion transmissibility of this infection associated with malignancy."[65] Dr. Roger Dodd corrected this quick assumption, reminding committee members that the highest prevalence of HHV-8 is in people diagnosed with HIV, not simply queer men.[66] Dr. Harvey Klein of the NIH went one step further, explaining, "We have transfused a lot of HHV-8 . . . and we really haven't seen an epidemic of disease. In fact, the CDC did some studies in the plasma recipients, the hemophiliac population, and really found almost nothing. In fact, they found nothing."[67] Driving his point home, he concluded, "I think we really need to remember that this is not transmitted very easily, not transmitted by stored blood."[68] With the window period for HIV depreciated, many in the group seemed to be looking for newly emergent viruses and assumed queer men would be ground zero for affliction.

THE IMPLEMENTATION OF SUSPECT EVIDENCE

The "epistemological dream" of science, according to Barbara Herrnstein Smith, envisions rational methods that cultivate evidence free of distortion, individual bias, social influence, and the "obscuring effects of sensory error."[69] Collecting "objective" data is a *telos* in itself and the credibility of scientific methods is often determined by the capacity to formulate seemingly non-subjective tools. Carefully crafted statistical models, examples that can be replicated, and facts presented as neutral all rest at the core of scientific logics. From the perspective of rhetorical deliberation, however, all evidence is inherently discursive, subject to the contingency of the situation, the cultural construction of classification schemas, and the audiences being constituted by or consuming the information. Proof is always prone to the interpretive nature of human beings. Methods of collecting evidence are fundamentally impacted by the presence given to variables, the subjectivity of the researcher, and those features omitted by scientific definitions.

The consistent turn to conceive queer men as embodiments of disease required a copious amount of evidence to underscore the excessive and intemperate nature of these citizens. Representations of disease were abundantly supported by problematic uses of evidence, reifying queer bodies as grossly impure and necessitating containment. The formulation of a diseased citizen in government meetings was not a simple matter of poor claims being inappropriately asserted. The BPAC utilized an onslaught of specious evidence to actualize their arguments against abating deferral policies.

Perhaps most shocking, much of the evidence used to track MSM infection rates and to predict donor conduct was derived from, of all places, STD clinical data. Pointing to one study, Doll pondered the implications of a map that sketched "HIV seroprevalence rates among MSM attending STD clinics in 12 cities in the United States in 1996." After surveying some of the data, she commented that it "is disturbing to note interestingly that in Seattle and Portland, nearly one-fourth of the MSMs with GC [gonorrhea/chlamydia] and nearly one-fourth of all [screened] MSMs in San Francisco tested HIV seropositive."[70] The fallacy in reasoning presented by the doctor is startling. Why is it disturbing to discover there are high infectious disease rates in STD clinics? A cornerstone of health and medicine is that people tend to seek treatment after problems have developed. Despite the best efforts of many healthcare workers, ours has never been a preventative system.[71]

To substantiate this slippery data, Doll presented findings from alternative studies that purported to track MSM behavior. She explained that younger men were sampled at public venues, including "various street locations, dance clubs, bars," almost apologetically stating, "so these are not STD clinics."[72] It is important to question the inferences that transpired for committee members when they heard variables such as "various street locations." Surely the evidence imparted visions of queer bodies in the cultural imaginary that fancies sexual behavior as always already illicit, transient, and prompted by substance abuse. While each of these could be radically productive for queer politics in other settings, in the hands of this committee the factors are both detrimental and irrelevant to discussions of queer *donors*. When placed next to FDA statistics finding that the average blood donor in the year 2000 was not "young" as described in the study, but thirty-eight-year-olds, this data is immaterial.[73] The rhetoric recreates a caricature of the promiscuous and irresponsible gay man by exemplifying stereotypical characteristics pitting sexual identity against conceptions of the good citizen. In this sense, "sex," not "citizenship" or "responsibility" becomes the master trope through which the discourse is constructed in the deliberations because the sexual act stands as the sole marker of identity. By marginalizing issues of citizenship and focusing specifically on sexual behavior, the committee altered the constitutive frame of community, as identity is suddenly located entirely in sexual acts (indeed, one sexual act since 1977) and those acts are never defined.

The conflation of queer blood donors and diseased bodies did not go unnoticed by some members of the committee. Dr. Mark Mitchell, for example, commented that "it just seems to me that there is such a disconnect between MSMs who are in clinics and those who might donate blood that it is hard to say anything, to draw any conclusions about the potential blood donors."[74] Rather than offer alternative data about the behaviors of gay men, Doll simply retorted, "Yes, and that is one of the reasons I mentioned it in the data limitations, knowing how much one can generalize from the clinics-based data is important. I wish I could give you that answer."[75] These "data limitations" were themselves glaring, but not scrutinized in the deliberation with the same ferocity that was given to the suggestion that queer men be allowed to donate. After discussing the clear articulation of disease and MSM for an extended amount of time, Doll offered an exceptionally brief disclaimer about how misleading her information could be: "Clearly, the estimates from the population-based data and the clinic data, I think we have to say they may not be representative of MSM blood donors."[76]

If queer patrons have any of the statistical similarities of the so-called general population of donors it can only benefit the blood supply. At the 2006 meeting Williams pointed out that blood donors, "whether they are first time or repeat blood donors, tend to be 10 to 1,000 times lower risk than the general population in terms of prevalence" for HCV.[77] Bianco added, "We should be aware that HIV prevalence in successful donors is lower than that of the general population, and not only HIV, HCV, HBV . . . prevalence markers among first time donors is much lower than that of the general population."[78] This promising news was one of the few times the civic potential of queer men was taken into account by the agencies. Still, there is no data that can sufficiently gauge donor rates until the ban is at least partially relaxed.

The locations from which much of the research on queer men was derived was equally important, as it called into question the scientific signifier "MSM" that tends to stand in for "donors." The interviews for Doll's second data set (the "various street locations"), for example, were not conducted just anywhere in the United States, but in specific locations that included Miami, Dallas, Los Angeles, and San Francisco. Each of these locations has typically been understood as having a sizable and visible queer community. In this light, the reliance on the term MSM becomes substantially less appropriate because the phrase implies an aversion to visibility and a retreat from political identity. For the BPAC, however, the vague and oversimplified phrase is used to define all male/male intimacy. As with the questionnaires administered at local blood drives, the scope of sex is never defined. Ironically, the acronym erases identity, behavior, and degree of same-sex experience, collapsing polymorphous practices into a single variant of subjectivity. Cindy Patton has elucidated the dangers of such thinking, observing that "even in the most elaborate gay theory, the process of gay identity formation is ambiguously articulated, and the role of sexual practice in gay identity is equivocal."[79] Dr. Steve Kleinman inquired about the problems of classifying a person who had one or two same-sex experiences over a decade ago in the same category with someone who is sexually active with men. Dr. Blaine Hollinger responded: "What you are getting into is the whole issue of what defines MSM behavior. That, in and of itself, is a complicated field. It is very hard to decide which of those two categories—if both of those categories are handled equivalently. We didn't have the data to distinguish between the two so we lumped them together."[80] Despite MSM being spotlighted as "complicated" the generalized term is never dismissed. This ambiguity is significant as it establishes differing standards for queer citizens attempting to make contributions to the community. Donating blood is a communal act, but one that is dependent upon individual responsibility to ensure the safety and well-being of lives. Rather than grapple with individual responsibility as it relates to civic obligations, the committee framed the discussion around the nondescriptive referent "MSM."

The decision to never define sex is a striking feature of these discussions. Despite the extended amount of time the committee devotes to poring over data sets, this most obvious of questions is hedged. "Sex," especially in queer communities, is notoriously challenging to delineate. How, for instance, might we define the moment a queer person loses her or his virginity? What sexual acts constitute this rite-of-passage? Must penetration happen? Does oral sex count? Are men who have never had sex with women, but only oral sex with men, virgins? Although not demarcating sex allows scientists to negate intimate details complicating an already cloudy quandary, this eschewing of definitions comes at the expense of positioning all sexual acts as innately dangerous. This understanding of disparate sexual practices as equivalent compels another risk. It subtly universalizes all sexual acts among queer men, failing to acknowledge that risk itself is at least partially constructed. It is well known that abstinence-only programs, for example, exacerbate risks because they take a universal approach to sex that ignores the convoluted relationship among sex, identity, and pleasure.[81] When blanket methods of defining risk are implemented and nuance disregarded, harms are more difficult to combat, not less.[82]

Time and again the committee downplayed the important relationship between questions of identity and behavior. One doctor explained at the 2000 meeting, the "question that we ask of persons who may have had sex with males as males is not do you self-identify as gay or bisexual. We ask, 'have you, as a male, since 1977, even one time had sex with another male?'"[83] Rarely, however, did their discussion escape the homosexual/heterosexual binary. For instance, comparing the risks between eligible and ineligible donors, one committee member noted, "but if it turns out [the behavior] is closer to the heterosexually active population, then it is not really changing the risk at all."[84] Unwilling to deal with the complex variations that stem from a diverse group of people, the agency clusters an array of populations together for the sake of scientific measurement. This strategy had dire consequences on the discussion, as it invited overt generalizations and stereotypical prejudices.

This mystification of queer sexuality with a seemingly innocuous acronym is rife with theoretical implications. In many circles "MSM" is often understood as being divorced from notions of gay identity in order to make judgments without implicating any one group.[85] Many men who have sex with men, after all, do not embrace the labels "gay" or "queer." Phil Wilson, one of the founders of the National Black Lesbian and Gay Leadership Forum and the National Task Force on AIDS has contended that the phrase "MSM" was actually developed by queer men of color as a compromise with scientific communities. He reflects, "Quite frankly it was a phrase that was created by black gay men, and we created it because we knew that the CDC would not fund black gay men."[86] In short, the phrase "MSM" can be a tool of political empowerment, not because it allows for new scientific stratifications, but because it refuses them.[87] In naming themselves, black gay activists could potentially take advantage of a system that has traditionally ignored, alienated, or abused them. Nonetheless, there is always the potential for exploitation. In official discourses, it is increasingly difficult to ascertain if dominant powers can now dismiss important cultural considerations, inspired by institutional neglect, by employing the nebulous phrase in their deliberations.

Gary Dowsett has contended the seemingly fluid acronym is ultimately costly for all gay men because of the erasure it yields. He writes: "Homosexual transmission of HIV becomes a simple variation in a unitary domain of *male* sexuality. This first, ignores the subordinate position of homosexuality and the struggle of gay men (and lesbians) to resist the structural relation between heterosexuality and homosexuality. Second, it obliterates from view the struggles of gay communities with the HIV epidemic and foolishly conceals the massive contribution of 'gay identity' and 'gay community' to their tremendous success at prevention."[88] The argument that the phrase "MSM" neglects important contributions made by LGBT organizations and activist groups in the fight against AIDS may well be true. Indeed, some have even suggested that the acronym has torn ownership of the epidemic out of the hands of the queer community.[89] While recognizing these limits, it would be wise to reconsider the claim that MSM presents no opportunity for making visible queer identities, especially in scientific discourses.

The phrase "MSM" holds vast potential for exposing the structural divide that is produced in scientific discourse. In the data about interviews conducted in Miami and San Francisco, for example, there is a clear nod to identity in urban areas where the studies took place. When researchers survey "MSM," they travel to locales where they know large numbers of sexually active men will be visible—the cities. In particular, it would seem that they are drawn to those places where people are open and honest about their sexuality in order to complete surveys and sampling, such as the aforementioned cities of Miami and San Francisco. So while it is tempting to assert that "MSM" remains apart from proscribed identities in scientific studies, the data used to produce the concept of "MSM" clearly indicates that queer life is closely aligned with this cleverly deceptive label.

In the past "MSM" has also been used to the detriment of queers of color in scientific discourses. One of the most famous cases of science instigating a discourse that had consequences for queer men is that of the "down-low" phenomenon. At its most simple, the down low refers to MSM who are frequently envisioned as also still having sex with women. More often than not, the down low has been associated with black men, even though men and women of all races conceal their sexualities and may have multiple sexual partners. More important still, the origin of the down low as a widespread practice and the subsequent HIV scare that ensued came not from the tabloids, but from the government. In early 2000 researchers at the CDC were attempting to explain why AIDS rates in some segments of the black community were on the rise. One researcher came up with the idea of the "bisexual bridge for HIV," blaming MSM of color for transmitting HIV to unsuspecting heterosexual women. The down low, however, has never proven to be a significant source of HIV transmission. Keith Boykin has observed that this theory burgeoned only with circumstantial evidence and deflected a number of important factors: that black women did not sleep with MSM of other races, that MSM actually had sex with women, that MSM were HIV-positive, that infected men were having sex with infected women, and that the sex itself was unprotected or unsafe.[90] To be clear, *no* study or series of studies have ever verified these links. And still the theory was asserted by a scientific community and spread like wildfire in the public sphere.

The evidence showcased here has been selected primarily because it played a central role in the discussions leading up to the decisions rendered by the committee. The ban was upheld in both years, and this problematic evidence was a part of the rational deliberative process that enabled exclusion. The definition, collection, and scrutiny of this evidence remain unchecked, receiving no attention from the press, other scientists, or even LGBT lobby groups. Its incorporation into the process is exacerbated only by the consistent uncertainties propagated throughout the talks.

A DISTURBING SCIENTIFIC PROCESS

The BPAC's rhetoric is even more problematic when one considers the ambiguous, fleeting, and at times overwhelming scientific process. The preponderance of studies on disease, most of which did not focus on blood donation, derailed the proceedings on numerous occasions. The lack of studies available on queer donors, coupled with the stigmatization of queer identity in favor of illicit sexual behavior, enabled the committee to delve into a sea of hasty generalizations. A striking characteristic of these transcripts is the degree of faulty and partial reasoning that relentlessly transpired. Even a cursory glance at the 2000 transcript reveals a number of logical fissures in the deliberations:

> "we *don't know,* in terms of exact numbers, what exact risk we are taking"; "*might* double or triple"; "we *estimated*" data in 1997; "*we do not have a complete but at least a better understanding* of blood-bank error rates"; the equation for determining numbers is "*really quite trivial*"; "because we want to be *conservative*"; "again, these numbers are pretty *iffy*"; "*could conceivably* contribute"; "We feel—we *don't have data to prove it*"; "These are very '*iffy*' numbers and, unfortunately, *it is all we have* to go with"; "some of the numbers here are *pure guesses*"; "But, again, that is *not the same as doing a good statistical analysis*"; "*There was really no evidence.*"

These are but a few of the analytical fallacies that jump off the page. The incomplete data and potential errors stand in sharp contrast to the definitive rubric created for queer men on donor questionnaires. The assumed ontological

force of queer sex is worlds apart from this flimsy development of epistemology.

Perhaps the most vexing question the committee had to contemplate involved the number of new queer donors that would give blood. The advisory
board frequently returned to the increase in contributions that would be cul-
tivated by relaxing the ban. Their statistics, however, originated with speculative comparisons to heterosexual donors and, as such, could not be verified.
As Busch explained to one media outlet, "They speak with certainty about
how many men would donate, the increased number of AIDS cases, etc. . . .
The fact is, they really will not know unless they test."[91] Even so, these statistically based assumptions were closely guarded. One doctor defended the estimates, asserting that "it is not all an assumption. It depends on what number
you are talking about because if it is the population number, the change in
population, how many new MSMs would present—that is not an assumption.
That was calculated."[92] Nonetheless, there was a significant gap between the
precise figures that could be calculated and the complete unknown. Queer
men had been deferred for seventeen years at that point, making any guesses
about increases in donations speculative. Even if one estimates based on self-
deferrals of queer citizens who do materialize in blood centers, there is no
distinguishing between the healthy donors and those regarded as ill because
their fluids were not harvested. Still, this clinging to an illusion of precision
was vital to many biased arguments.

Continually, the doctors are baffled, stating "the question is going to be
how can we quantitate this," or "I am not sure how to quantify it."[93] As such,
many committee members found it difficult to discuss queer men outside the
rubric of the vaguely calculated "MSM" paradigm. For example, one member
asked if the number of men who regularly test for HIV had been examined
in any of the studies being used to make conclusions. This question confused
the presiding doctor, who replied, "we do have a number for what frequency
of men who donate have a history of deferrable MSM behavior. We do have
that number, but I am not sure what you are looking for beyond that."[94] The
likelihood that many queer men *who donate blood* monitor their bodies and are
health conscious is seemingly absent from the process.

Sadly, not all prejudice is so unconscious. Even within the confines of a
scientific forum an explicit turn to outdated, injurious stereotypes was present. A letter read at the second meeting from the leader of the military's blood
collection organization, Colonel Eugene Fitzpatrick, managed to touch on a
number of bigoted labels. He claimed, "MSM is a known high-risk behavior
and, while there [are] those donors who have changed their lifestyle, they are

relatively few and . . . these donors are not always truthful."[95] The colonel asserted that rethinking the deferral policies was nothing more than a political ploy, continuing, "We know HIV is transmitted by transfusion and yet this risk is acceptable because individuals *choosing an alternate lifestyle* are being discriminated against."[96] In a space littered with subtly discriminatory evidence, the candid letter, if nothing else, at least revealed the ubiquity of politics and prejudice in the deliberative process.

To be fair, a number of committee members raised important questions in opposition to overgeneralized claims or unfounded evidence. During the 1997 meeting, for example, Mitchell reinforced his skepticism about the data brought to the table regarding STD clinics. He "was very disturbed by the usage and the comparison of some of the data for the highest risk people in STD clinics . . . saying that there is no difference between them and, let's say a monogamous male couple."[97] Likewise, Martone objected to a conflation between new diseases, emerging infections, and queer men, arguing, "I don't think you want to restrict it to MSM. I think this is also a problem of heterosexuals, of children who don't have sex, and a large segment of the population."[98] He also reinforced the necessity of using data that details the number of men who have tested negative for HIV in the last year. Further, Hollinger called into question the allegation that queer donations would cause a tidal wave of new infections because of the amount of blood collected from the twelve largest U.S. cities. As one doctor stated, an "awful lot of the blood that is collected doesn't come from cities, and we know . . . that the relative rates of MSM are three to four times as high in major urban areas as in nonurban areas."[99] These objections not withstanding, the doctors arguing for a relaxing of the deferral policies were not offered the same consideration as those opposing it. Pollution, it would seem, is always easier to construct than purity in the scientific process.

Although these individual concerns could indicate a thoroughly examined understanding of MSM behavior, the number of arguments considered by the group left the subject of sexuality distorted and dangerous. The sheer amount of data presented to the committee became an issue during the discussion. Dr. Joel Verter implored the BPAC to ponder the harmful conclusions being produced by the preponderance of evidence under review. He argued, "Oftentimes we are presented with a volume of data at the meetings which, to say the least, they are overwhelming and almost impossible to correctly interpret in my opinion. . . . A lot of this data was based on many assumptions."[100] The avalanche of statistical and scientific data is especially problematic when one considers how it garbled the relationship between sexuality, disease, and

identity. The following exchange between Dr. Jane Piliavin and Dr. Hollinger
at the first meeting is representative of the perils of data overload:

> Piliavin: "I want to get back to this prevalence issue. It is also not just the
> possible mixing up, but someone raised the issue of needle-sticks, and
> so on, with the health workers, and if it is indeed the case that some-
> thing like 70 to 80 percent of men who have sex with other men
> are positive for hepatitis B, that is an awful lot of possibilities there.
> Again, I would like to see something like what Dr. Martone . . ."
> Hollinger responds: "Jane, it is not that high. I mean if you look at high-
> risk age group, it has been 80 percent with hepatitis B markers, which
> is usually only somewhere between 5 and 15, or maybe 4 to 15 per-
> cent may be HBs antigen-positive. It depends on the population."
> Piliavin: "All right."
> Hollinger: "But when you are dealing with the people who might come
> in and donate, then, the markers fall down to maybe 40 to 60 percent,
> and again, of those that are probably infected, it is probably closer to
> 4 percent or somewhere in that range."[101]

The amount of data collected by the committee, distributed in written form,
and then verbally clarified still did not help to sort out the abundance of material the members had to consider. Here was a doctor who had been framing
70–80 percent of all queer men as positive for hepatitis B for hours as she was
presented the rest of the information to make an "informed" decision. Voting
to relax the deferral policies is almost unimaginable from such a standpoint.

Despite these failings, the committee found ways of reinstituting the
treacherous and wild nature of gay men. Consider the convoluted assertion
put forth by Piliavin, the same person who made the erroneous miscalcula-
tion about hepatitis above. She argued:

> One of the things statistically about the sexual behavior of men who
> have sex with other men, of men who have sex with women, and of
> women who have sex with men, is that the number of partners of people
> in those three groups is highly statistically significantly different. So, if
> you think in terms of a person presenting who says I am in a monoga-
> mous relationship, and this person really does believe that they are in a
> monogamous relationship, that is, they know they haven't been having
> multiple sex partners, it is still statistically the case that if that person is
> having sex with a man, then, the likelihood is that it is of a much higher

likelihood that if the person having sex with a man, that the partner is indeed having multiple partners, and that is multiplied if it is a man having sex with a man, simply statistically on the basis of what we know. So, the question of people who claim they are in monogamous relationships, who are men who have sex with men, is still more problematic just on the basis of what we know about these groups of people.[102]

Queer men can never win in these discussions. The evidence lodged against them is always contorted to represent them not as civically oriented actors, but as a stereotypically irresponsible (if not hostile) group that is a threat to the blood supply. Here one finds the deflection of blame from queer men to "men," but queer men are always doubly damned when understood in this light.

Not surprisingly, the committee fell back on the image of the queer man in denial of his afflictions with some doctors arguing that such people are deluding themselves. One of the BPAC members contended: "They don't intentionally try to mislead you because they don't ever get to that point, they have convinced themselves that even though they may have engaged in these behaviors, it is okay because, and they don't really mean me, because, of course, the person I had sex with couldn't possibly have had a disease, and so on, and so forth, those kinds of things, so there is inherent problems in this question."[103] In this statement one finds the extreme of Foucault's *scientia sexualis,* with state officials literally mapping the thoughts of the imaged queer man into the deliberations. There is no need for the voices of actual people in this monologue, as the statistical and empirical data provided all of the necessary narration. She failed to inform the committee about the degree to which high-risk behaviors across *all* age groups, races, sexes, and sexualities were increasing.[104]

As the government continues to extend its biopolitical tendencies, it is imperative to continue "queering" scientific deliberation procedures that infuse the language and logic of institutional voices, further fragmenting queer communities while rendering self-serving classification schemes possible. Because donating blood is not a civil right, tied more explicitly to social acceptance, civic identity, and rhetorics of purity, the BPAC's reasoning must be stretched to its rational limits. The creation of policy based on questionable scientific processes that essentialize queer men because of their lack of civic virtue or supposed sexual excessiveness must be combated. The state persistently invokes science to uphold the blood ban, but other blood collection agencies are speaking out against the exclusions. Competing findings from organizations such as the ARC are opening up new possibilities for donation privileges, but such work is rarely given consideration over state-sponsored data.

While several committee members expressed dissatisfaction with the manner in which the blood-donor screening question is worded, they also refused to alter its language. At the day's end they sided not with those who are being discriminated against but with the system.[105] The ban stands to this day. The deliberations narrowly constructed sexual identity as located in the sexual act alone, even as such acts remained undefined. This construction of sexuality devoid of cultural and contextual variables was significant as it reproduced several malicious social constructs of queer men.

BLOOD MONEY: HIDDEN TRANSCRIPTS OF CAPITAL

One would be remiss to think the FDA is unmarked by politics, economics, and social pressures. Busch, a strong advocate of lifting the ban, noted that "there is a lot of political and, if you will, public pressure to not relax the gay deferral."[106] Even in the realm of science, there are always political presumptions that require scrutiny. I spent ample time attempting to verify a quotation by one member of the committee who asserted he had an obligation to "be in compliance with the publicly mandated and congressionally mandated policy of zero error tolerance in this matter."[107] Importantly, there is no such congressional mandate. That power, along with the imperative of the unmarked heterosexual public, was assumed.[108] Despite this fictive assertion, it illustrates the strong tie between science and the state that many people fear.

Although masked in the transcripts, there are significant economic pressures steering the proceedings. Indeed, if cultural identity received scant attention from the committee, economic considerations were left unspoken. One should not lose sight of the fact that keeping blood safe is a costly endeavor. When the move to cleanse the blood supply was made in 1985, Patton questioned if the motive was entirely benevolent, explaining, "'Bad blood' may be 'bad business' for this major U.S. industry."[109] A decade later, in 1995, the BPAC voted down a test that would have detected HIV within days, but came at the cost of $30 million. Fortunately, a key government official who was ethically troubled by this action forced the measure through and had most members of the committee removed.[110] Jean-Jacques Rousseau's musing that public finances are the blood of the social body is especially appropriate here.[111] To lift the ban would require additional tests, new questionnaires, and no doubt a public relations campaign to ensure the "general public" that giving and receiving blood was still safe.

These economic considerations subtly permeated the meetings under examination, with important portions of the deliberations gently insinuating the economic and legal questions the committee confronted. References to cost were scarce, but occasionally surfaced in telling moments. Bayer was one of the few doctors to mention cost in any of the forums. He alluded to the fact that all blood could be tested repeatedly for donors who incited concern, but costs prohibited such possibilities.[112] Revising questionnaires, testing their accuracy, and sampling blood require an immense expenditure of capital, and those expenses often fall to organizations like the ARC. Nonetheless, as one doctor pointed out, the true impact of altering the deferral policies "won't be known unless we understand what a revised question might do."[113] It is not surprising that the ARC refused to mitigate the ban at the first two meetings.[114] The organization strongly opposed *any* change in the decision to allow queer men to donate blood. In the ARC's view, "The patients that we ultimately serve [must] be our number one policy. Second, it is a public-health issue, not a social policy issue."[115] Despite the influence of the ARC and the force of their arguments, the organization insisted they were powerless in the debate. When asked if they would be open to the possibility of moving to a policy that would defer queer men from giving blood only if they had had sex in the past five years (still omitting numerable healthy patrons), one ARC representative offered the following response: "Our questions for deferral are based on data that were presented to the FDA by the CDC. The practices that you are now talking about and the population studies have not come up with an increased risk to the extent that this risk behavior does. So, if the CDC were to come to the FDA and say 'I have a new practice and it is obvious that this is a high risk practice, we need a question,' we would be the first to accept that."[116] The reasoning was tautological. No conclusion can be ascertained about queer donors until they are permitted to give blood. However, the ARC insisted that data must first be collected before they alter the forms. This may be a reasonable stance on the part of the ARC, but it also permitted all the organizations involved in this debate to blame others for the deferral policy instead of proactively working to change it. Busch criticized the ARC's stance, saying: "Your proposal says wait until we have the data, how do we get the data until we can do studies in the context of revised questionnaires? A proposal that says wait until there is data to address these things is basically saying don't address changing them ever because, until we have a mechanism to implement studies—the measurement is right there."[117] Antonio Gramsci reminds us that civil society attempts to remain "legally neutral" and "exerts a collective pressure and obtains objective results in the form of an evolution of customs, ways of thinking and acting, morality, etc."[118] It is easy to understand why one critic asserted that it "seems likely that money, marketing, and sheer arrogance are factors contributing to ARC's maintenance of the policy."[119] At the same time, if the BPAC will not advance similar considerations and continue to hide behind diseased images of queer men, they can hardly cast stones at the benevolent organization.

The above dialogue notwithstanding, economic considerations were chiefly erased to preserve the rhetorical purity of blood. The ARC, which always has a voice in the BPAC meetings, generally divorces issues of money from public discussions of blood and blood donation. They were one of several national blood organizations that spoke out against awarding blood-drive contracts to high-bidding collection banks when one center wanted to offer twenty-dollar scholarship funds for each pint collected, but then sell the fluids for two hundred dollars.[120] It remains vital to organizations such as the ARC that blood not be constructed as a commodity.[121] To constitute blood as a commodity renders it impure. As blood is the defining mark of the social body, it is necessary to keep it both sexually and rhetorically cleansed. Even more important, as long as blood is understood as a service, and not an item, lawsuits against the blood industry are almost impossible to pursue. Just as Foucault has suggested that the "accumulation of men and the accumulation of capital—cannot be separated," here the corralling of volunteers who feel civically and ritualistically pure is central to a vibrant blood business.[122] When these organizations rhetorically purify the blood of the nation, they not only marginalize economics, they decisively scapegoat "polluted others" to reassure citizens in the "general public" that they are both special and secure. If there were greater economic incentives for the blood industry, if they needed more bodies for increased profits, perhaps such ferociously stigmatizing images would not be present in this rhetoric. In the 1997 transcript it was suggested that lifting the ban would present a less than 1 percent increase in the amount of fluids collected for the blood supply—hardly a substantial gain. The benefits simply did not outweigh the projected costs.

But businesses are always looking to the future. With the advent of NAT and strides in LGBT rights, organizations such as the ARC began to shift their stance on contributions obtained from queer men. Bianco, who represented America's Blood Centers, warned scientists at the 2006 workshop that the collection agencies were losing young donors because of the deferral measures and their practices could be impeded for decades. Bianco reported: "Many of our centers are unable to collect blood, particularly in colleges and in other environments, because of a perception, and a real perception by many of the students, that we are being unfair about the issue that has been discussed all day today, that is, we have different criteria applied to different risk groups, and people don't understand the risk groups. These issues impact on our donations."[123] Bianco implored the scientists to rethink the policies, saying a one- or five-year deferral would still incite problems. "It would not address

the perception of discrimination, so would not resolve the social, political issue associated with these deferrals."[124] Although the issue of blood donation
has not gripped the media, it has been taken up as a cause by young people on
college campuses and in high schools. While most blood drives attract new
donors at a rate of 15 to 30 percent, in high schools and on college campuses
this rate rises to 80 to 100 percent.[125] An entire generation of potential patrons was at risk because of young people's commitment to equality.

Since the initial meetings the ARC has spoken in favor of altering the indefinite ban against queer citizens. The benevolent organization now argues
for a one-year deferral policy for sexually active men, putting the onus back
on the BPAC to lift the ban. The ARC has forcefully asserted that "the current lifetime deferral for men who have had sex with other men is medically
and scientifically unwarranted."[126] As the web site at the start of this chapter
reminds us, science's powerful voice will likely be the one that ultimately al-
ters these stigmatizing practices. This institution will also be the one that re-
assures the general public that giving and receiving blood, even with queers in
the midst, is safe. Until then, the people most likely to challenge these prohibitions are queer men who both pass to donate blood and protest in the ritual
space. Those citizens, fighting to change the system, are considered in the next
chapter.[127]

5
Passing, Protesting, and the Arts of Resistance
Infiltrating the Ritual Space of Blood Donation

The act of donating blood has long symbolized an altruistic relationship of connectedness among citizens in a polity. Almost universally regarded as a volunteer endeavor, giving blood is a simple deed that takes little time and effort, usually in places of communal import. As a performative act of civic engagement, blood donation functions simultaneously as an intimate bond between strangers and a public ritual that affirms civic identity. Blood donation is, to borrow Michael Warner's phrase, an "intimate theater" that constitutes publics and shapes minute dimensions of subjectivity.[1] In the everyday performance of citizenship there are few occasions when people are hailed to express their commitments to strangers in the polity. The explicit avowal of civic identity in the ritual space is an exception to these silent, "deep rules," executing an illocutionary force that materializes identities.[2] Blood donation is especially noteworthy given that "democratic citizenship requires rituals to manage the psychological tension that arises from being a nearly powerless sovereign," generating trust and sacrificial reciprocity among anonymous citizens.[3]

When confronted at blood donation centers with inquiries about sexual history there are two clear ways for queer men to answer. The first is to openly admit that they had participated in acts that run contrary to the safety standards adopted by the Food and Drug Administration. In the ritual space of public sacrifice they may confess their "sins" and either protest or withdraw quietly. The alternative is to deny their sexual history, roll up their sleeves, and allow their symbolically tainted blood to flow into the bodies of six strangers living, or perhaps dying, in the polity. Lying would reduce embarrassment, avoid confrontation, and dismiss the institutionally mandated exclusion. On the other hand, if the men are caught, it could lead to disciplinary measures, depending on the motives of the contributor and the quality of his blood.

These dastardly options motivate the twin modes of resistance—"passing" and "protest." Which mode of resistance, one might ask, should queer men select when confronted with a choice between lying and self-condemnation? Which is the more productive mode of dissent and opposition: passing or protesting? For all of their heterosexist implications, these invasive procedures are effective only to the extent that citizen actors obey them. The Blood Products Advisory Committee may draft reprehensible documents that position queer bodies as threatening, but only queer men can affirm such conceptions during the screening process. By passing, queer men can penetrate the system and reaffirm their ability to survive in a world that regards them as impure. But by verbally protesting, they can initiate debate and discussion with blood center workers that could instigate change within collection organizations.

On its face, it would appear that queer men lie to donate blood, or alternatively refuse to hide their identities, because they wish to be included as "citizen equals" in the larger polity. While such a reading could be potentially advantageous in a culture where the term "equality" carries considerable cultural capital, these understandings address only one aspect of a complicated rhetorical situation.[4] Equally significant is the fact that queer men choose to pass, or refuse to lie, in order to defy reductively ascribed notions of identity. They resist a state-sanctioned, predetermined essentialism by refusing incorporation into neatly defined categories of classification. While so-called identity politics is often critiqued as a brash form of activism that falls into the hazardous throws of essentialism, serious work remains to be done on those factions which are always already positing all queer men as essentially the same.[5]

In this chapter I argue that "passing" and "protest" are correlates of one another, existing not as two separate strategies, but as reciprocal forces that attempt to enact social change.[6] Although passing may not always appear resistive, its importance as a mechanism of pride, power, and moral agency should not be ignored. As James Scott has noted, "So long as we confine our conception of *the political* to activity that is openly declared we are driven to conclude that subordinate groups essentially lack a political life or that what political life they do have is restricted to those exceptional moments of popular explosion."[7] Indeed, comprehending the necessities of *infrapolitics* is central to understanding the social resistance of oppressed groups. Robin Kelley has argued that infrapolitics and verbal resistance "are not two distinct realms of opposition to be studied separately and then compared; they are two sides of the same coin that make up the history" of activity among marginalized people.[8] Probing the connections between men who lie to donate blood and those who refuse to deny their sexuality offers new insight into the factors that motivate each group, the self-negotiations they make, and the discursive violence enacted on their bodies.

Conceptualizing those forms of daily life not always visible to power structures, what Scott refers to as "hidden transcripts," is easily accomplished using contemporary understandings of passing. However, when addressing issues pertinent to the blood ban, it is difficult to ascertain the significance of passing without contemplating the verbal protests of queer bodies in the ritual space.[9] The men that protest demand recognition as members of a diverse collective not easily stereotyped and excluded. They are motivated by the systemic harm inflicted on them and, as a result, resist culturally ascribed generalizations. They do the important work of reminding blood collection agencies that they are a constant presence in the polity—and that where one of them resides, there are assuredly more. The significance of these contestations are striking in that they not only articulate a refusal to pass, but also affirm the very *potential* to pass.

Just as protesting draws attention to practices of passing, so too does passing support discourses of dissent. Passing affords the men, in the words of Charles Morris, an "obscured agency, and immersion in the mainstream, precisely so that one might swim against the tide, undermining the homophobic order of things."[10] The men who openly dissent draw attention to those who pass and, in doing so, force questions about the number of queer donors and the amount of "tainted" blood slipping into the system. If one takes seriously the claims made by the FDA that blood donations from queer men would lead to heightened infections in the blood supply, then the logic follows that gay men who give would spark countless problems. Knowing that there are men who have sex with other men who continue to contribute blood should present evidence of increased infections. Such has not been the case.[11]

This chapter critically analyzes the responses of twenty-one men I interviewed to explore how "passing" and "protesting" function in this ritualized space. Their experiences are an important, but often overlooked, aspect of this discursive and political battle. Importantly, none of the men who has given blood has received notification that his blood has been discarded, was tainted, or has gone unused. In short, their blood is as pure as the fluids of any heterosexual donor. This infiltration renegotiates everyday sociality with the knowledge that "intimate relations and the sexual body can in fact be understood as projects for transformation among strangers."[12] The men in this study initiate discourses that are subtle and often unseen, but are also slowly gaining attention among blood collection agencies, college students, and citizens eager to invoke change.

PASSING AND PROTESTING

The term "passing" is generally regarded as the ability of a member of a dis-
enfranchised group to render "invisible" those traits used to oppress them
culturally and institutionally. Having eluded aspects of gender, race, class, or
sexual orientation, people can paradoxically live their lives more openly when
occupying a privileged space of secrecy. In Anna Spradlin's account, "'Passing' is how one conceals *normal* information about oneself to preserve, sustain, and encourage others' predisposed assumptions about one's identity."[13]
Such actions have the potential to subvert traditional notions of identity and
belonging, creating new forms of identification, opportunity, and difference.
Passing can "represent viable means of survival and self-transformation under
conditions that temporarily limit . . . moral agency."[14] These practices fashion a
public subject who is momentarily empowered by a rearticulation of identity
generally assumed to be transparent. Passing blurs insider/outsider relationships by rendering indistinguishable those normally positioned as "we" and
those typically demarcated as "they."

Passing is especially significant to theories of identity as it approximates the
degree to which performance is an intricate element of the self. Elaine Ginsberg notes that passing is inherently performative as it is "neither constituted
by nor indicating the existence of a 'true self' or core identity," while simultaneously being "bound by social and legal constraints related to the physical
body."[15] The "passer" takes advantage of cultural codes of performance to
redefine abstract notions of the self in concrete and material ways. Passing is
dependent on an audience that can be "duped," a set of circumstances that
facilitates the means of specific performances, and an agent capable of executing the pass effectively.[16] Its discursive specularity (or lack thereof) sparks
opportunities and anxieties, replete with rewards and penalties.[17]

As a historical phenomenon, passing has been employed to scrutinize the
machinery of performance in quotidian life. In a world where queer visibility continues to balloon, it may seem counterintuitive to suggest passing
remains a necessary tactic of survival. However, passing maintains its relevance
in many facets of LGBT life, especially those emanating from cultural institutions that stress solidarity, sacrifice, and ritual.[18] Passing facilitates the creation
of purified identities in ritual settings where notions of kinship and stranger
relationality are not always equivalent. The U.S. military, for example, actively
encourages soldiers to pass. Queer personnel must render their bodies "pure"
through silence about their sexual orientation. While the shadow of AIDS
shades this debate, the more common justification for the "don't ask, don't
tell" policy centers on troop morale and unit cohesion. The visible incorpora-

tion of queers in hierarchical arenas imbued by rituals violates the heteronormativity keeping their sacrificially docile bodies "pure." Similarly, in many faiths those who perform rituals dependent on discourses of sacrifice and purity must be both male and avowedly not queer. Blood donation has long depended on discourses of purity to substantiate claims to safety, which is why volunteer blood is always more desirable than purchased fluids. The ritual site constitutes these common understandings of sanctity and pollution.

While passing is not as openly defiant as traditional forms of protesting and certainly digresses from the standard mantra of "coming out" as a dutiful aspect of politically motivated principles, it can be an empowering experience, one that allows marginalized groups to avoid the "obsessive classification" of institutional bureaucracies such as science.[19] Catherine Squires and Daniel Brouwer point out that "passing is a transgression that inspires fear in the state and dominant social groups" because marginalized groups are usually contained through codified knowledge and systems of control.[20] Despite such advantages, there is an ambivalence to these critiques. They maintain that while passing has the potential to cross boundaries, it also has the power to reinforce traditional categories between identity groups. Such conclusions surface frequently because passing is usually studied only after a person's normally assumed identity has been historically revealed.[21] However, passing also facilitates particular performances of stranger relationality.

Although passing is generally understood as challenging social norms, it is seldom understood as a viable form of performance that reinforces and dialogically fortifies existing conceptions of stranger relationality to strengthen community. Passing does more than draw attention to the inauthentic nature of identities. In the rhetoric of the blood ban, passing illustrates how all performances are unstable, all identities are inherently constitutive. This realization is not an impediment to communal bonds. Recognizing that citizenship is a signifier forever in process is the driving force of stranger relationality. Passing, like protest, seeks inclusion in the power structure, but questions the arrangement of the network it is challenging with the hope that "the poesis of scene making will be transformative, not replicative merely."[22] Both the men who lie about their sexual identity and those who express their orientation in this study, for example, are motivated by a shared need to exist in a diverse polity. They are moved by an audience that has instilled in them the value of community, the need to resist oppressive discourses, and the necessity to take their stories of transgression back to the communities where they reside.[23]

Those who cover up their sexual experiences in order to give blood are able to demonstrate firsthand that they are not vessels of disease longing to thwart the body politic. They occupy the ritual space of blood donation in a manner that allows them to resist universal notions of queer sexuality by attaining scientifically mandated clearance that they are in fact "healthy." They give their blood, it is tested, and when they are not contacted about negative results, their gift proves the contentions of the protestors. Passing reclaims and then reconceptualizes institutionally developed understandings of queer bodies, helping to disarticulate those identities from conceptions of disease. The men prescribe a personal antidote to the vexing plague of medicinal generalization and in doing so reconstruct their roles as citizens.

By protesting at the site where they are denied access to a ritual of citizenship, queer men also have the opportunity to alter the system by expressing the dangers of stigmatization on a local level. While such overt resistance inevitably prohibits them from participating in the act of blood donation, these men recuperate their citizenship by invoking dissent as a form of civic engagement. In short, they reject the implication that they are impure. Rather than reiterate rituals that reinscribe heteronormative identities, they rupture traditional notions of citizenship by disrupting the reconstitution of imagined purity.[24] With little more than their personal experiences to assert their arguments of purity and desired civic inclusion, they introduce the important claim that they should not qualify for deferral.

Protesting generates opportunities for publicly ruminating about the numbers of queer men donating blood. While organizations such as the American Red Cross carefully avoid public controversies about discrimination, the agency is bending under the weight of protests. On rare occasions it acknowledges that people of all sexual orientations have either withdrawn from donation or ignore the rules completely. At a 2006 meeting about deferral policies an ARC spokesperson told the FDA that universities and colleges are increasingly protesting blood drives and that "many individuals with deferrable risks continue to donate."[25] The presence of protestors incited concerns about the number of people passing. Shortly following this presentation, a student organization called "Fight to Give Life" enlisted more than twenty schools to protest in blood drives nationwide. A gay man leading the effort noted, "I lied when I first gave blood, at 17, because I was afraid to say 'yes.'"[26] Collectively, they are creating change: the ARC now opposes the FDA's stance on indefinite deferrals. While strangers lurking in the "hidden transcript" are not visible, their practices reverberate in the public sphere where policy is being negotiated.

In both passing and protesting, queer men constitute themselves as citizen actors. In defying the mandate of the FDA (quietly or loudly), these men return to their communities and develop stories of resistance with family members, friends, coworkers, blood donors, and others who share in their ongoing struggles. They are ordinary people becoming narrators of their own lives, defining "the (common) place of discourse and the (anonymous) space of its development."[27] These networks of resistance are rarely publicized, but have an important influence on the integrity of the men and the agency they achieve in partially constructing their roles in the polity. This discursive circulation allows them to "fashion their own subjectivities around the requirements of public circulation and stranger sociability."[28] Although the deferral policies often compromise the manner in which queer men understand their bodies and civic identities, their actions remain a rich source of civil disobedience.

I turn now to the interviews conducted with twenty-one men who have, on some level, participated in the ritual act of blood donation.[29] I share their stories to illustrate the diverse ways in which queer men perform their citizenship in a ritualized space, even as institutional mandates strive to control the process and outcome of that performance. Their experiences represent the ways in which passing and protesting can act as weapons of the weak. These donors give presence to the fact that queer men are ever present in the body politic and that their contributions and motives are far more diverse than otherwise imagined by advocates of the blood ban.

CIVIC IDENTITY AND GIVING THE GIFT OF LIFE

Whenever a group of people discuss their experiences, there are few places where the word "always" is useful. While several men expressed a civic and national obligation to donate blood, others were deeply conflicted about having to "pass" and consciously self-excluded at the donation site.[30] Some men easily voiced the concerns they had with the blood ban, while others had a difficult time articulating what troubled them so deeply about this particular form of exclusion. Many of the younger men had never lived a day without the blood ban being federally enforced, while some of the older men had been donating since well before the word AIDS was uttered for the first time. Despite demographic differences, the civic act of giving blood was always tied to personal norms of communal obligation. Like Danielle Allen, these men understand that sacrifice "makes collective democratic action possible."[31] Many of them noted that donation was important because blood is an irreplaceable substance with no known substitute, but one that is exceptionally easy to harvest. Some asserted that they gave blood because people they knew were deferred as a result of health conditions. Still others said that collection agencies were missing out because they were the highly valued "universal donor."

The impulse to give blood to reaffirm communal identities was strongly illustrated by the first man I interviewed, Adam, who has given blood in a number of locations where he has lived in the United States and England. As a citizen he saw it as his duty to donate blood in the communities where he resides. He reflected, "If you can do something as little as a pint of blood, why not do it? I think that as a citizen, you're someone who participates in a community, good or bad, you're there." Simon, who refuses to donate blood on the grounds that he has to lie about his sexuality, furthered these thoughts on citizenship. "I think of myself as a citizen," he said, "as someone who plays an integral part of society, meaning the everyday kind of operation of being a part of the community and then having a voice in our local, state, and national policy-making machinery." He added, "When I was younger everyone was told you should be giving blood and then you get into high school and you have all these blood drives and you're made to feel bad if you don't because it's like you're participating in something that's essential. And, you know the same thing happens when we have a local or national crisis . . . whether it's a Mother Nature kind of thing or whether it's [a] terrorist attack."

The social pressure to take part in blood drives described by Simon should not go unmentioned. It is frequently noted by both queer men and the scientists who dictate the deferral policies that social pressure is a common reason for wanting to contribute.[32] All recognize the potential the ban has to contribute to feelings of isolation and stigmatization.

The desire to participate in the civic ritual of blood donation often stemmed directly from personal experience. Many of the men had personal motivations for donating, and these reasons often took precedent in their minds over national identification. Family members who had suffered illness or injury, for instance, regularly surfaced in the interviews. As Simon explained, "I think for almost everybody, including me, at some point it hits home that someone in your family needs blood." The coupling of necessity and family often gave way to conversations about familial rituals. Bartholomew, who used to volunteer countless hours for the ARC, commented that his mother could not donate blood, so his father often did. "I think that the fact that my father donated a lot of blood made me feel like I should continue with it." Thaddeus's memories of blood donation are directly tied to an annual family event. "There's one crystalline experience in my memory growing up where my parents' church always had a blood drive the day after Thanksgiving. And it was just this thing where everyone went together." Caleb felt even more strongly about these health issues because he benefited from a blood donation as an infant. "I know that when I was born I needed a blood transfusion. And if I ever decide to have children or anybody in my family needed blood, I should be able to give it to them." Although not going so far as to call it a right, the attention to family indicated a particular ethic of care stemming from norms of communal obligation and personal ability.

The association between blood and kinship is self-evident enough in the previous paragraph. What is striking is the idea that donation is something nearly impossible to imagine outside the bonds of community. It requires a reflection on the permeability of human life and the dependence people have on one another. The men recognized that "an environment of strangerhood is the necessary premise of some of our most prized ways of being."[33] Time and again, the men reaffirmed ethical impulses constructed from the most basic units of the social order—their partners, parents, friends, and local communities. As Jacob noted, "For me it really is a part of responsible citizenship and . . . there's this need clearly out there that you hear about all the time. . . . People need blood and it's not something I can do, and no one can really tell me why I can't do it in a way that makes sense to me or in a way that feels fair." The injustice here is not simply directly at the donor, but the anonymous recipients in the polis who benefit from a surplus of liquid life.

Catherine Bell reminds readers that it is in the ritual act that people constitute themselves as citizens.[34] Prohibiting access to civic rituals can contribute to the depletion of associations between notions of the self and conceptions of an engaged citizen actor. Regardless of their decision to give or withhold, this symbolic import did not go unnoticed by many of the men. Blood donation articulates a unique relationship between the donor and the community in which she or he lives. Matthew noted the special significance of giving blood. "There are other things to get involved with in the community, but I think giving blood . . . is like giving life. I feel like when I'm giving blood I'm helping out in a medical sense. Certainly, if I were in need of blood I would hope that there would be enough supplies that perhaps I could have some of it." So powerful is this constitutive element of citizenship that several of the men had a difficult time identifying other equally meaningful acts of civic participation. While some thought giving blood was parallel to volunteer work, and a couple aligned it with voting, most thought the ritual act of donation carried a distinct cultural capital. Philip said that one *could* compare giving blood to volunteering, but the analogy trivialized the importance of donating. "I just think that giving blood, it kind of goes beyond that. You know, you're helping society, you're helping yourself, I mean you never know a year down the road when you're going to need blood, so you know all those other people who are doing it too. I think it goes a little beyond a right to vote or volunteer time." Likewise, Matthew struggled to verbalize the feelings he had about blood donation, pondering it for several minutes, repeatedly trying to offer an explanation. "There's something about being able to give blood that's a little different than just volunteering your time. And I'm not really sure how to put that into words beyond that. But, it's more like—recycling life." It is this ambiguous constitutive power of blood donation that makes it so admirable. More than a simple exchange of fluids, it captures a civic relationship that implies interconnectedness, sacrifice, and ultimately life.

The exclusion from performing these identities prompted a number of men to comment on the ways in which they understood their citizenship to be systematically corroded. There were more remarks on the role the ban played in positioning the men as second-class citizens than all the other comments collected. Andrew, for example, bitterly noted that "I have had people ask me, they have the little sticker that says something like 'be nice to me, I gave blood today' and they ask 'oh, did you give blood today' and I'm like 'no, they won't take my blood' and it makes me feel like it's the 1960s when they didn't want to take black blood and mix it." Philip picked up on this segregation metaphor, arguing, "It separates a certain section of society and it puts them in a corner saying, 'You're not good enough' or 'We don't agree with your lifestyle.' It just puts us in a little box. We fight every single day not to be put in that box." Bartholomew explained, "It's awkward when people ask me, 'are you donating blood' and I have to tell them 'no.' And I feel at times— especially after the attacks on the World Trade Center—I felt like I was being anti-American for not donating."

Many of the men also observed that the ban is given considerably less attention than other issues advanced in the LGBT movement. One of the respondents had been involved with a state Human Rights Campaign organization and was told by group leaders that the blood ban was simply a "minor issue" compared to gay marriage or adoption. However, he was never certain if that really meant it was a more difficult issue to broach. In a similar vein, Thaddeus said that the issue was more complicated than others he had encountered. "I think I have moments of, 'this is just one of those battles that I just haven't picked.' This is just one of those things, like anything related to gay men and AIDS that I'm not going to win. . . . I'm just going to scream until I'm red in the face and it's not going to go anywhere." Paradoxically, the ban is rendered less significant precisely because it is a decisively more arduous issue.

These men embraced the communal obligation of blood donation as more pressing than suspicious generalizations. Being excluded encouraged feelings of isolation and alienation. The cultural capital of this ritual, coupled with emotional exclusion, often led many of the men to lie in order to donate. Passing afforded the opportunity to disprove false claims advanced by the institutions mandating the ban.

THOSE WHO PASS

One of the biggest fears the FDA exhibited when they first implemented the blood deferral policies was that hordes of gay men would donate out of spite, disdain, and vengeance.[35] Although several of the interviewed men continued to donate blood despite their contempt for an agency that condemns them, all professed altruistic motives for their sustained donations. Indeed, the lack of overt political motivation was almost disappointing for those who study counterpublics and their resistance to state mandates. Passing was regarded as a necessary evil for aiding other citizens. It was also a means of protection in locations where they could be "outed."

The blood ban has varying effects on the way queer men understand their place in the citizenry. Despite the strain these policies can have on the men who pass, each of the people who lies in order to donate blood serves an important function when one contemplates resisting the ban. The men create alternative narratives about their health and the productive impact they can have on their communities. In giving voice to these experiences, the donors forge new possibilities for challenging the ban, articulating "hidden transcripts" among those deferred. When the men in this study detail their experience it aids in disproving the disparaging policies sanctioned by the government.

By passing and then verbalizing their stories, the scandalous donors are able to give firsthand accounts of why the current policies are out-of-date. All of the men interviewed have shared their stories with other people—family, friends, and coworkers. Each has contributed to a discourse of dissent in opposition to the FDA and blood collection agencies. In doing so, they create communities where struggles are mediated outside the reach of those in power. They generate new forms of identification and gradually build discursive means of resistance. A quick survey of their responses illustrates this well enough. Adam, for example, insisted that numerous queer men he knows lie to give blood. "They feel that it doesn't matter, that they're not participating in high-risk behavior, so it's not an issue." Isaac said when blood drives come through town he often shares stories of donating with other people, particularly gay men. Philip has spoken to most of his family and friends about the deferral policies. He explained, "I think everybody that I've talked to about it thinks it's extremely unfair, discriminatory, that certain members of society are singled out . . . just because of their sexual practices." Likewise, Peter said that he talks about the guidelines with other people every time a blood drive is held at his workplace. Paul has led chat-room discussions on the Internet with gay men about the blood ban and many were unaware that it was in effect. More often than not, men who pass tend to complain to family and friends about the discriminatory rules. Aside from Paul and his web-site discussion, most of the men confined their exchanges to people with whom they are close. Regardless of the limitations on their conversations, it is important to note how these men dispute overgeneralized harms associated with queer blood by placing their bodies in the ritual space to disarticulate notions of disease, enabling new understandings of citizenship and communal responsibility. Despite the lack of media attention given to this issue, for example, the demonstrations held on college campuses emerged through everyday networks, not large-scale organizing.[36] Scott reminds us that the "hidden transcript is not just behind-the-scenes griping and grumbling; it is enacted in a host of down-to-earth, low-profile stratagems designed to minimize appropriation."[37] The prohibited donors reposition their stigmatized identities and put forth small initiatives on behalf of fellow citizens in the polity.

The resistance calibrated by these men is striking when one contemplates how often they have donated with no reports of infected blood. Despite scientific accounts that depict queer bodies as contagions, these men push against the long-standing theme of living in social denial discussed in earlier chapters. They create a space in the ritual site that excludes them, simultaneously forging relational bonds with others receiving their blood and resisting the discursive images of disease constructed on their bodies. These men all stated they gave precisely because other citizens were in need of blood and they had the resources for providing it, even as some attested to a desire to avoid being outed. By recognizing the limits of their identities as queer men in these situations, they initiate new forms of moral agency. The prohibited donors productively reposition their stigmatized identities and put forth small initiatives on behalf of fellow citizens in the polity.

The men who digress from the policies are able to foreground the role of citizen as their master trope of identity and discount elements of their sexuality often constructed as threatening. Isaac, for example, asserted that the question simply did not comport with his way of life. He explained, "I take into consideration that they're not taking into account my lifestyle. . . . I've got perfectly good blood. Why should I be turned away or discriminated against just because they have one question in there that bans other people?" The need to make a difference was often attributed to the frequent blood shortages and the lack of people who regularly donate. Bartholomew gave just over a gallon of blood in a short amount of time. "I just felt that the benefits out-weighed any risks I posed. I felt like it was one thing I could do that some people had difficulty with. Usually you can make due without certain services—you can't make due without blood." John continues to contribute blood in large part because it is one of the small ways he can give back to the community with his busy life. "Look, I'm a forty-year-old man. I'm never going to have children. This is my way of contributing to mankind's good."[38] Only one man, Andrew, said that being subversive was specifically on his mind when he donated—and even that was only part of the equation. "The first time I was like 'well, I can't do it' and then I just decided to do it because it doesn't matter. I don't know—I was kind of rebelling, I guess. I wanted to do something so I lied and maybe that was wrong." Each of the men believed that the exclusionary policies were misguided and as citizens they had a duty to disregard the measures that were created in opposition to their identities. This disavowal of the question is significant in that it illustrates a new understanding of the power of passing. While passing is often positioned in academic literatures as a mode of individual empowerment, here it can be looked at as a productive form of building civic relationships. While queer men undoubtedly get personal satisfaction from the donation process, they are also privy to the idea that they may be saving the lives of one or more individuals.

From a critical standpoint, the interviews also offered the opportunity to examine an array of important issues regarding the body and cultural politics. One of the more compelling phenomena that transpired during these discussions was the common theme of "being caught." A number of the men felt they could be "outed" by blood collection volunteers. From their perspective, such forcible revelations about their identity could result in unknown punishments from the state. Adam, the man who had given blood in England, recalled his first experience with the intrusive questionnaire. "I just said 'no' and I just prayed that they couldn't tell." He believed that blood center officials could discern that he was lying from his pulse and blood pressure. "I didn't know if they could even assume that you were gay and say, 'You can't donate.'" Peter had a similar experience. He reminisces, "I remember reading that and thinking, they're going to know. I got teased a lot about [being gay] growing up and somehow I just thought they would know, even if I answered 'no.' I guess I was waiting for so long for someone to really call me out on it." Paul said the first time he heard the question he was completely caught off guard. "I was even sweating at one point I was so nervous. Every time the nurses came up, I kept thinking they were going to come up and say, 'We saw the way you were looking and we want to talk to you a little more.'" This fear of literally being called "out" demonstrates how the intrusive question furthers feelings of isolation and alienation. The men were attempting to aid the community by providing an irreplaceable substance—but were instead introduced to the very site of the discursive reiteration that energizes the construction of "the other." They recognized the power of that constitution and the role they play in sustaining the demarcation between "us" and "them." These anxieties were especially pronounced in their reflections on the law and its relation to the deferral measures.

Five of the men who stopped lying in order to donate blood brought up the consequences they might confront if they were "caught." However, none of the men could cite the punishments they might face. Thomas, for example, said he did not want to deal with the legal repercussions that could accompany lying, but he had no idea what those might be. John also brought up the legal aspect of donation and confused lying on the stand in court with the questions he responded to at the blood donation center. "What's the legal term when you lie? Perjury? I figure that the Red Cross and the National Bone Marrow center could possibly, I don't know, bring up perjury charges or something." Paul wondered if he could be taken to jail for denying his sexuality. He pondered, "If they found out I was sleeping with men, have I committed some sort of perjury? Or they'd put me on some list somewhere."

This vague image of legal repercussions is striking insofar as the men did not need to know the punishments prior to disciplining themselves.[39] Although gay men will be turned away for admitting they have had same-sex experience, it is difficult to prosecute a person for lying about his sexuality unless he knowingly contributes to the spread of a disease. Further complicating this ambiguity, some organizations such as the American Association of Blood Banks have established so-called hearsay rules. So, if a gay man donated blood, a third party could report his donations because of his "high-risk" status. The AABB would then call him and ask if he was in fact a member of that high-risk group. Regardless of the answer, the blood is often discarded. After all, proving that a person is in fact queer would require much investigation, and collection agencies traditionally avoid such tactics.

However, Paul was not wholly mistaken when he expressed concern for being placed on a list. For instance, people who violate any of the ARC policies and are caught, or who admit to not being eligible to donate blood, do have their information recorded on a list. This information is stored in a database that can be accessed by ARC volunteers in specific regions.[40] The list is not specific to "men who have sex with other men," but to all people who must refrain from contributing blood. Matthew was the only man who said he had literally been "caught" giving blood when he was not supposed to. The healthcare professionals were very polite, but very direct—he was not to contribute again. Although curt, the ARC took no other actions to ensure he refrained from attending blood drives in the future. "They didn't threaten any action. They just basically said, 'You can't do it.' If you come back in again, your name will be on a list or whatever and we won't take it." The projected fear of reprisal is usually enough to keep men away, but this literal monitoring is troubling for citizens eager to participate in blood drives or those concerned with privacy issues.

This surveying of the body hit especially close to home for one of the men who was confronted about his sexuality by a blood collection worker. John was "outed" by a coworker who reported him to the ARC. He recalls: "I got a phone call from the Red Cross and . . . it was from the blood center and she said, 'I understand you donated blood at work last week.' And I said, 'Yes.' And she said, 'Well, we got an anonymous tip from someone who says you're a gay'—how did she put it—'a practicing homosexual.' And I almost said, 'Honey, I don't need any practice.' But I didn't, I played it very straight. And I said, 'No, that's not true.'" Despite the encounter, John continues to give when they hold blood drives at his place of employment. In fact, the phone call secured his donations well into the future, precisely because he wishes to conceal his sexual orientation at work. If he stopped donating, his colleagues could easily confirm he is gay. The ARC refused to disclose who had tipped them off.

Often the question furthered thoughts about exclusion in the community for the men who were not yet at ease with their sexual orientation. Several of the men were in the closet when they first attempted to donate blood. Because many of them were not "out," were married, or had limited resources for exploring their sexual orientation, they were caught off guard by the query. This frequently influenced the way queer patrons understood their identities in relation to others. Paul explained that he was married when he first started having sex with men. It was during this time period that he began to donate blood. "I got that sick feeling in my stomach. I was kind of shocked when I read that, actually. There was a part of me that thought I shouldn't give, and then a part of me that was thinking I should get up and walk out, but that would be even more obvious. I'm married with kids." Being in the closet can be a treacherous period of time for LGBT people. Some people never fully "come out" and those that do still face discrimination and abandonment. Despite all the resources available, coming out of the closet remains a difficult and frightening time of life for many people. The current policies of the FDA do little more than add to that fear of exclusion for these citizens. Matthias, for example, said the question "stunned" him. "Part of it was I was in the closet at the time. It was just more of an embarrassment than anything. I don't even know how to explain the feeling—just like that 'ugh' feeling, that nervousness, almost like you're just turning red. Honestly, I just didn't expect to be asked that question." The discomfort guided these men to reiterate an identity free of nonnormative markers that render them impure in the ritual space, furthering feelings of isolation.

Being closeted was especially difficult for people who came from small towns, where much of the nation's blood is collected. Because blood drives are often housed in places where many townspeople gather, and because the volunteers are more likely to know the donor, answering affirmatively to "are you a man who has had sex with another man" is simply not an option. In some locales these questions are asked orally and reinforced with written documents. Thaddeus, for example, donated where his parents worshiped. He relayed, "I remember thinking, 'my God this just happened where my parents went to church. I was more embarrassed by the other people in the room. . . . Then I was thinking, 'I suppose it's a necessary safety measure, blah, blah, blah.' I think I was a lot more self-hating at that point. I remember thinking I was really singled out." Matthew also gave blood in his hometown church for the first time. He lied in part because there was a pressure not to be discovered by the people in his community. He recalled, "I had been with a guy. . . . The church and these people knew me so I wasn't going to say 'yes' anyway. It was a really small community of like maybe a thousand people in the whole town at that time and there are like five churches. But I knew these people really well and they knew my family quite well and I wasn't ready for that yet." Already combating an unusual amount of surveillance, the questionnaire did little more than initiate anxiety and reproduce feelings of insecurity for citizens who lived in small towns or rural areas.[41]

For a number of the donors, living "out and proud" is simply not an option. Among the men I interviewed, at least two had specifically mentioned being members of the armed forces. Their stories are especially intriguing because of the conflicting policies at play when the military sponsors a blood drive. Since the early years of the Clinton administration, the "don't ask, don't tell" policy has supposedly guaranteed job security to those who identify as gay or lesbian.[42] Under such measures, the military is not to inquire about a man's or a woman's sexual orientation (though queer people are constantly investigated without just cause). When collection agencies appear on bases to collect blood, however, such direct questioning does transpire for queer men.

Blood drives are common occurrences on military bases. According to the servicemen, the ARC can show up multiple times in any given year. Because so many people in the military are either trained to give back to the community or carry heartfelt notions of altruism, the armed forces are an excellent source for generating donations. Awareness that members of a community might soon need blood seems especially pertinent in military settings. In order to collect as much blood as possible, the blood drives are often construed as spirited competition for the women and men serving. Units compete with one another to collect the most blood and wear the accomplishment as a badge of pride if their troop is successful.

Isaac recalled the first time he ever donated blood was while in the Marine Corps. He donated between twenty and twenty-five times while enlisted. "Back then it was probably more like, can we get more than this unit … in our entire unit of seven hundred people, because not everyone would actually qualify because of the locations troops were sent to. It was a competition that would benefit other people." But, he noted, there were occupational benefits to contributing blood as well. "At the beginning the impetus was 'go down and give blood get the rest of the day off.' So, it was just a reward for giving blood. I think it turned into 'hey, this is something that's good' and I continued to do it. It's just something that's developed into a sense of giving back to the community."

Philip said that the blood banks would regularly visit the military base he was on and they were always warmly received. The competition to donate blood was good natured and often a morale booster. "A lot of times we'll have one squadron that will compete against the other squadron and it's just kind of for bragging rights, and you know, you get people involved and I think it does encourage people who may not be as willing to give blood or have a lazy attitude about it." Philip had always enjoyed providing blood, but donating on military bases was awkward because he had to verbally deny his sexual orientation. "I think the first few times when I donated blood, I felt guilty for saying no because I knew it wasn't true … but I just continued to donate when I felt I needed to." This bind not withstanding, neither Isaac nor Philip regretted their donations.

The situation faced by these men offers an intriguing cultural loophole. Legally, they are entitled to refrain from divulging their sexuality by way of the "don't ask, don't tell" policy. In fact, because people with viruses like HIV are not permitted to serve in the military, many of the questions contradict military standards. Of course, the men could always withhold donation during these drives. But to do so potentially calls into question their sexual orientation. How many times can a soldier hide behind the guise of being afraid of pain? How long before the loyalty to their unit is questioned? Their willingness to give should be valued, not anxiously contemplated.

Not all men are willing to make such sacrifices. Several of those interviewed felt the need to protest overtly the actions of the FDA and blood collection agencies. Much like those who pass, they have a felt obligation to retain a sense of dignity, but do so by refusing to lie. They believe there is integrity and pride in embracing those elements of their identity used to position them at the margins of the polity.

THOSE WHO PROTEST

The most endearing and amusing stories came from men who were confrontational with the people turning them away. When asked "are you a man who has had sex with another man," seven of the respondents refused to conceal their sexual orientation. These men insisted they were safe in their sexual practices, had been tested for HIV, and had every right to be treated as their heterosexual counterparts. These men refused to "pass" in the name of "the public." Rather, they forced conversations about sex, blood, and altruism. They felt that the diversity of the queer community was oversimplified in the FDA's policy, their contributions as civic participants were disparaged, and their relationships maliciously denigrated.

Protesting the policies is significant because it confronts cultural archetypes about queer men being universally HIV-positive and posing a greater threat to the polis. Acts of verbal digression force reconsiderations of civic identity about those who are included and excluded in cultural rituals. The importance of producing this space—one which clearly posits queer citizens are not impure—is vital to the resistance calibrated against the ban. When these men protest, they advance the claim that they are safe in their sexual practices and have a desire to be a part of a community regardless of damning policies. In doing so, they invite an important question—are they really disease free? Dialogically, if one recalls that none of the persons who has lied has been told he is harboring infections, the contentions of the protestors illustrate that the FDA has little evidence to support the assertion that queer blood is contaminated.[43]

Most of the men who refused to lie did so to resist the institutional sanctioning of insidious stereotypes. This dissent occurred in many forms, including people who have repeatedly fought institutional generalizations. Simon, for example, attempts to give blood on a regular basis, even though he recognizes he will be turned away. "Even after I knew I wasn't supposed to, I did it just to make a point." Simon, who works at a university, says he reports the ARC to the GLB incidents team each time they come to collect blood. "It got really irritating for me, particularly because it was as if something that I was doing was dirty and nasty and yet some of the students that I work with all the time that I know really well, you know had had five or six sexual partners in the past two weeks. And I've had the same sexual partner now for eight years. Why that's seen as negative, I don't know." Simon regarded it as his duty to report the ARC to the harassment team because of the potential effect it could have on students. "The first time I just left. I felt totally rejected. After that I became vigilant, I just went, completed it all, then the person told me that I couldn't [donate] and I complained to them about it." According to Simon, the ARC agreed to post signs at blood donation sites to save students the embarrassment of being asked the invasive question, but the organization rarely follows through on this promise. He was especially troubled by the fact that the ARC was encouraging students who were banned from giving blood to help out in other ways, such as working the table where cookies are served to other donors.

Protests often transpire during moments of crisis, when the reiteration of a definition, characteristic, or identity is called into question. While crises often galvanize political unity and sacrifice, the necessity of defining who one is at times of moral uncertainty can have a powerful role in the constitution of self.[44] A plethora of the men said they showed up to donate blood at an important juncture in their lives—immediately after coming out. In contrast to the men who lied because they were not yet "out," these donors, having recently struggled with the uncertainty of their sexuality, could not in good conscience conceal their sexual orientations. Jacob, for example, rebuked the policy at a time in his life when he was frustrated with a world that forced him to deny his orientation. So, he defiantly told the blood center workers that he was gay and disappointed in their measures. When he first attempted to donate years ago before sexuality was so openly discussed, he said it embarrassed the volunteer. He describes her as having a "bright red face." He remembers, "I mean every time. Regardless of whether going through the screening or debating or talking about the issues, 'where do you now stand on this,' it's always the same—bright red face." Similarly, the issue of pride motivated James to confront a worker. "I went up and said, 'What's up with this?' You know of course I was young and a college student. I was probably pretty irritated by it. Obviously they weren't going to give me the answer I wanted to hear." In this defining moment, proclaiming his newfound sense of self was most important. Despite the lack of immediate change to the policy from these individual contestations, the collective weight of these encounters is paying off. The ARC's break with the FDA is evidence the benevolent organization fears losing young donors forever because of negative associations established early in life.

Denial was considered deleterious by many of the men, as it conjured up images of the past when they were trapped in the closet. Jacob indicated the ban made him feel like a second-class citizen in much the same way being in the closet can feel personally oppressive. He was uncomfortable with the "whole concept of denying who you are. . . . I want to be afforded the opportunity to do that without being harassed on the way." Mark concurred with this notion, saying this policy infringed on his quality of life because of the misconceptions it circulated. He explained that when he thinks of the blood ban "the first thing that comes to my mind is that it feeds into other misconceptions and instills fear." In this case, that fear is that all gay men are living with AIDS and carelessly harming others. Simon matter-of-factly contended, "I think it just ties into a lot of other ways that as a gay person I'm invalidated, dehumanized." These feelings of being implicated in the cultural imaginary as treacherous actors, however, instigated many of these men to act—not be passively interpellated.

Protesting illustrates a desire to break free of institutional approval, even as it simultaneously seeks affirmation. All of the men who admitted to having sex with another man did so primarily because they had no interest in passing, no pressing need to fulfill altruistic needs in a manner similar to the men who lied. At the same time, they expressed bitterness and sadness at being excluded. The sacrifice of blood donation is supposed to feel good, not produce disdain and contempt. Mark never thought his sexual orientation would be an issue, since he never had unsafe sex. Of course, he was still turned away. He recalled: "After I came out I was involved in a relationship. And when I came out at work and everywhere else I decided I wasn't lying anymore. So, during one of the blood drives at work I was asked the question, 'have you ever had sex with men,' and I answered, 'yes.' And that was when they stopped the interview and said I can no longer give blood." Mark participated in a heated argument with the blood-drive worker, who told him he would be indefinitely deferred. "My response was, 'Wait a minute, you didn't ask what kind of sex I had or whether it was protected.' . . . I remember saying, 'Are you asking me oral sex or anal sex?' And she just got kind of all bent out of shape. She just got real nervous. She was uncomfortable with my honesty. . . . And I remember saying to her, 'Are you asking me if I've ever had unprotected sex or not, and the answer to that is, no, I have not.' But, you know, again it was if you've ever had sex with another man." Mark's experience is not an isolated incident. Answers are rarely offered to men who dispute the measure at local blood centers. The bureaucratic hierarchy lodged between those deferred and those who produce the regulations is one of the most difficult problems facing individuals who oppose the policies. While HIV/AIDS activism can often be pursued on the community level, such is not the case for the blood ban because the policies are regulated by national organizations. Protests illustrate the lack of responsiveness to inquiries and the omission of relevant data to mandate the deferrals. Often, center workers and volunteers know little about the ban or have no control over its reach.[45] Andrew, for example, says he became politically active in the funding for AIDS research and was hoping to make a small difference when it came to the deferral measures. He responded:

"I was starting to get more politically involved with a lot of different things. So I went in, not really to donate, if they had accepted me I would have done it, I just wanted to ask them about it. And they gave me the policy, they were a little abrupt and short with me, and they were like, why was I questioning it? 'This is based on sound medical standards' and I tried to point out that these were not sound standards at all." But to no avail, there was no change in policy. Andrew was prohibited from donating blood and little more was accomplished than upsetting the blood-center workers.

The inability to justify the ban is especially baffling in regards to civic identity. While the donors who are deferred seem to contribute blood because of communal obligations, and divulge pages of personal information to do so, they are simultaneously denied an extended rationale for the existence of the policies or access to the people liable for crafting the measures. Those in power are safely positioned "off stage," privy to their own "hidden transcript" of domination. Blood-center workers occasionally presented an ambiguous government or civil society hierarchy to the men protesting, but none of the deferred donors was given answers that addressed his questions about personal responsibility or safe sex.

These deferred men articulate a decisive link between queer men and their abilities to be engaged citizens resisting inequitable policies. By withdrawing from the process they interrupt the assumptions of the state, insisting that the "purity" of this ritual is deeply tainted. They question the fear of difference, pointing out that generalized claims always fall short of the diversity of men who have sex with other men. Rather than assimilate, they remain abject, constituting otherness, but always reminding those at the blood centers of the failures inherent in their blanket typification. Understandably, some will argue that these men simply give the system what it desires—a segregation of queer blood. But one should not underestimate the narratives these protests could provoke, the people they could influence, or the attention to passing it affords.

Sharing such protests is not only vital at the site of the ritual donation but also in the larger polity. This is especially true when one contemplates the number of men who are encouraged to conceal their orientation. Several of the men who refused to lie reported that friends and family often questioned their willingness to disclose their sexuality. More often than not, people told them to simply cover-up their sexual orientation. James, Mark, and others made a special point to say that lying is simply not an issue for the gay men they know. Many of their friends lie, give their blood, and continue with life. Mark frustratingly recounted, "Everyone that I've ever shared [the experiences] with has always said, 'Well, why did you tell the truth' or 'Why did you tell them,' both gay and straight people I know. They all lie." For men like Mark the reiteration of an identity based on lies pollutes not the blood of the nation, but the bonds of the communities in which they live. They should not have to misrepresent themselves.

Although most of the men were strongly discouraged by the ban, it should be noted that some were not convinced the policies were related to citizenship. For example, Thomas believed the ARC had no right to enforce discriminatory policies, but he did not feel they necessarily imposed on him as a citizen. This, despite the fact that Thomas organized a blood drive at his place of employment after a natural disaster and over six hundred people donated because of his efforts. It was at this very location he discovered he was not able to give blood. Thomas was not "out" at work and the very blood drive he set up to aid the community became a site for keeping him in the closet. While he was exceptionally proud of the amount of blood collected, he still wished he could have donated. On a positive note, he observed, "There was no way I could have given six hundred people's worth of blood . . . so, at least I still did something good." When Thomas approached a gay and lesbian civil rights' group about the ban, they simply chalked it up to an issue they could not win. He was told it was "a minor issue in comparison to everything else" that the group was fighting for, such as antidiscrimination laws in housing, employment, and adoption. The omission of the blood ban as a significant issue, and one less imperative than standard civil rights struggles, illustrates the importance of dissent produced by queer men. Pressure has not been applied by national and state organizations as much as it has everyday citizens who feel maligned in this dastardly rhetoric. But, when citizens take up the cause, they do not necessarily see the connection between queerness and civic identity. Like the groups that are meant to represent them, such matters are generally reserved for issues inscribed in law, not in vernacular culture.

Both the men who pass and the men who protest are resisting scientific and cultural projections of their bodies as contagious basins, continually redefining their capacities as citizen actors. Nonetheless, the blood ban still engenders several poisonous effects. It encourages these donors to understand their bodies as less immune to sickness and harm than their heterosexual counterparts. While there is strong potential for resisting the ways in which the policies impose themselves on queer men, these donors still fall victim to harsh generalizations promoted by the FDA.

THE RECALCITRANCE OF RESISTANCE

Queer men recognize that these policies are based on grossly distorted scientific data used to malign them. However, simply because the policies are resisted and self-evidently biased does not mean they have no impact on queer men or the ways in which they understand their bodies and conceptualize their civic identities. Indeed, the deferral policies created a number of problems that prevent any romanticizing of these resistive practices. One of the more distressing findings of this study, for example, was the degree to which queer men expressed doubt about the health and permeability of their own bodies. In many ways, they became strangers to themselves.

Most of the people who stopped donating said that they did so because there was always a fear in the back of their minds that somehow, somewhere, things had gone wrong. A condom had broken during sex. A new virus strand would be discovered. They had placed too much faith in science. They had not put enough trust in their doctors. Continually, they positioned themselves as potential threats to the very strangers they were hoping to aid. Despite the felt need to pass or protest, the ban altered the way many of the men viewed their bodies. Bartholomew, for example, was concerned that scientists might discover some new strand of HIV and it would eventually be traced to him. "Morally I thought, okay, maybe they don't know enough about this, who am I . . . and I just thought maybe I don't really know enough about this to go against top-notch researchers." Although confident in the safety of his own sexual practices, the disciplinary arm of the state penetrated his mind. He never considered that many researchers oppose the deferral policy.

The articulation between HIV/AIDS and queer identity constantly surfaced over the course of these discussions. In the face of the claims made by the FDA that gay people are not implicated in these policies, the men consistently called into question these establishment assertions. Although significant strides have been made in HIV education, a number of people continue to view AIDS and being queer as synonymous, and this includes a number of gay men who live in fear of their own sexuality because of these debilitating connections. This is not to say that queer men cannot be infected or that danger to the gay community does not exist. But these blanket declarations mask the productive role queers could play in society and the dangers presented by rhetorically purified categories of health risks to heterosexual communities. These interviews revealed a continued hierarchy in the fight against HIV/AIDS, with these men believing themselves to be more susceptible to disease (regardless of precautions) and more predisposed to hurting other people.

Thomas stumbled over his words as he attempted to express why he had stopped lying in order to donate blood. "Fear of—if I were to be an HIV carrier—that someone else would contract it and then I personally would know they contracted it." Philip shared these concerns, saying, "I think in the beginning it was the fear of 'oh, gosh what if I did give blood and it came back positive.'" He continued, "I had always practiced safe sex and so I've never worried about that, but there's always that doubt. There's always that thinking, 'oh Gosh' maybe there was that one time I slipped up." Paul insisted that he never felt as though he was a member of a high-risk group sexually, but the deferral policy called that certainty into question. "Every time I gave . . . I had that fear still that I might get a card that would say, 'You need to call us.' There was still that initial gut fear that when I gave, I would get a letter that said 'you're positive,' or whatever, and 'why are you giving' and I'd go to jail or something." While he donated frequently when he was experimenting with oral sex, he explained that he only gave once after having anal intercourse. Despite being tested for HIV, he still felt a substantial degree of guilt for days after giving. "At that point I knew I was at much higher risk, even though I was using condoms, I still felt I was at a much higher risk than I had been. . . . The fear was that by doing this I could really hurt somebody." Although Luke had planned to withhold donations for political reasons, he also began to question the degree to which his sexual activities, all of which he described as safe, could overpower the blood supply. "I consider myself very low risk, most studies would say no risk. And once that changed then I started reconsidering, 'what do I want to do about this.' Obviously, nobody wants anything bad to happen." But precautions were often not enough to convince many of the men who were not carriers of malicious agents.

Often, this self-doubt tied directly to their identities as gay men. Bartholomew was actually angry with himself after he came out and discovered he could no longer give blood. He sadly recounted, "Because of my decision to have sex with men, I now lost the opportunity to donate blood. . . . There were many times that I questioned my sexuality, you know, all that I potentially had to lose by engaging in a gay relationship and I thought well here's another way I lose that." He later commented, "I remember now, it was more like 'oh fuck, here's another way gays have screwed up,' it's just fuel for the fire." Thaddeus had similar thoughts: "I just remember it was pretty soon after having come out of the closet and I just remember thinking, 'these are the things gay people have to worry about and this is your life now,' a kind of 'this is your life' moment." Regardless of personal responsibility, safe sex, or limited experiences, all nuance is lost to "this is your life," a peculiar euphemism for discrimination and hardship.

Resistance here may appear to be compromised, but one should not undermine the important function of self-doubt in creating a mode of self-empowerment. Shame often constitutes the very identities people embody.[46] It is, as Shompa Lahiri reminds us, the active policing of the boundaries of identity that "thrust private acts of transgression into the public domain and in the process laid bare the hidden spaces of identity formation."[47] The system may have an effect on queer bodies, but that does not wholly negate resistance to the system initiated by the men. Nonetheless, it is not surprising that a large percentage of donors had grown discouragingly ambivalent toward the policy.[48] Their pride is chipped away, often encouraging them to focus not on the well-being of the polity and the advantages of donating healthy blood, but on their bodies—whether diseased or not. Thaddeus remarked that he had grown up in New York where there were constant blood shortages. He had a difficult time comprehending why they omit so many healthy donors. "I don't think of it in terms of like a right to donate blood, like, 'you need my blood more than I need to give it.' So like, you can have my healthy blood. My type of blood is AB negative, it's useful. Fine, don't take my 'gay blood.' It's one of those stupid things." This attitude that queer men would defer themselves was shared among some interviewees. "I guess after the first time . . . I was like, if you don't want my blood, fine, I'm not even going to try. So, you're missing out." Remarks such as this are reminiscent of Julia Kristeva's observation that "indifference is the foreigner's shield. Insensitive, aloof, he seems, deep down, beyond the reach of attacks and rejections that he nevertheless experiences with the vulnerability of a medusa."[49] Repeat donors are typically people who have a heightened understanding of the needs of the community and their own bodies. Here, however, it is easy to witness the dilapidation of communal bonds as the corpus of the other is rejected.

Such indifference is troubling when one considers that people's lives are at risk when perfectly good donors for blood, or other substances such as bone marrow, are omitted without just cause. Joseph had his only experience with deferral policies while he was attempting to act as a bone marrow donor. He says that he had registered while still in college. About four years after graduating he received a letter from the registry saying he was a potential match for someone in need of a transplant. In the letter, however, they included a reminder about who was eligible to donate and who was not. "So I called the number and told them that I didn't meet the qualifications since I was gay, and asked whether they still wanted to test me. They said no, and that was the end of the matter." Discovering such a match is exceptionally rare and there is a strong possibility that a person may have died because of a negligent and prejudicial policy.[50]

This disdainful situating may contribute to another disparaging effect in which some men felt the need to establish hierarchies of healthiness in opposition to other citizens. Women, for example, came up frequently when discussing groups that were allowed to donate.[51] While some remarks were more institutionally supported than others, there were a number of remarks that compared gay men who could not give to female donors who could. While specific examples of populations that should not be able to give blood were never solicited, various respondents were quick to offer illustrations. Isaac, for example, was comparing a monogamous man to a sex worker in one instance, arguing "a female can come in—a female prostitute who sleeps with you know twenty, thirty guys a month can give blood with no problem." Likewise, John and Andrew brought up the image of the "prostitute" and complained about the ease with which they could contribute blood.

To be clear, sex workers are not supposed to donate blood. The forms clearly state that if you are a person who has sex for money, you should not give blood. However, these frequent remarks were striking not simply because of their misogynous tendencies, but by the obvious need to constitute a "lower being," someone so absolutely impure by virtue of her sexual habits that she is in need of even more stringent regulation.[52] Regardless of the intent, the men interviewed almost always returned to the image of the female body for comparison to their own. While there were references to "heterosexuals" broadly, and these images remain largely without gendered explanation, more specific examples clearly identified women. Philip, for example, remarked, "I may be mistaken, but my understanding is they can ask a woman if she's had seventeen sexual partners in the last week, but she can still donate blood." Philip is not completely off the mark with this speculation, as the FDA asks women only if they have had sex with a member of a "high-risk" group recently.

Of course, there are not likely to be many women who have seventeen sexual partners in the duration of seven days. So why did several of the men tend to employ this imagery? One answer might lie simply in the patriarchal structure of our culture. After all, they may be gay men, but they are still men. The image of the female body as more polluted, more excessive, and more dangerous is a long-standing trope of Western history. Or, perhaps these comparisons were drawn because both heterosexual women and queer men have sex with men. To avoid totalizing, there were several positive references to women throughout the interviews. For instance, Luke thought that gay men could learn from the feminist movement, especially when arguing that small, quotidian details such as language choice are important. "Look at the feminist movement and lots of the issues they raise that people would never have thought were disempowering." These affirming remarks were especially abundant when considering the amount of good things many of the respondents had to say about blood-center staffs, overwhelmingly composed of women.

Indeed, the gender composition of blood-center workers may be at the very heart of this stigmatization. A large number of the men who were confronted, turned away, or forced to lie were screened by women. Here one finds another harmful outcome of a policy that is devised by people who are never in the position to turn donors away from giving blood. It is entirely possible that the structure of blood collection organizations like the ARC, having so many female volunteers at donation sites, engenders a situation in which queer citizens connect their deferral experience with a female citizen. As such, the shunned donors are repeatedly creating arguments in their heads to prove their worth, refuting those people who essentialize, stereotype, and ultimately dismiss them. It is one more way in which organizations that mandate the ban are able to draw attention away from their policies and onto the bodies of unsuspecting and essentially powerless strangers.[53]

The idea that some blood-center employees themselves might play an important role in allowing queer men to give is intriguing. After all, people who work for blood centers are limited in their ability to prevent gay men from donating. One blood-center worker told me she has witnessed a number of gay men donate, but does little to stop them. Adam recalled an experience where a member of a blood-center staff outright acknowledged the number of donors who were gay. He was recounting his first blood donation experience to the worker who was playfully inserting sexual innuendo into his story. "I said, 'Michael was the first guy that did me when I came in' and I didn't mean it in a sexual way but she was playing around and she was like, 'You know you shouldn't tell me you're having sex with guys,' and I was like, 'I never said that, but even if I was, I wouldn't be donating here anyways.' And she said, 'Everyone does it, it doesn't matter. They're all breaking some rule.'" It was obvious to Adam that the blood-center employee knew he was gay. But he simply had to say "no" to the question on the form and there was little or no follow-up on this inquiry. A number of fascinating questions arise from such seeming recognition. Did the blood-center worker still use his blood? How often do such occurrences transpire? Or perhaps most important, did the volunteer identify and sympathize with Adam's desire to donate blood? Like all people, blood workers are subject to their own opinions based on their own personal experiences and relationships. While I did not directly interview blood workers, it would be wise not to overlook the fact that many people, like many members of the BPAC, do not agree with the deferral policies.

STRANGER RELATIONALITY AND
THE RECONSTITUTION OF "BAD BLOOD"

Blood donation secures its value as an imperative cultural practice only to the extent that strangers repeatedly actualize the discursive bonds of public life.

The urge to resist pain incurred by the puncturing of one's skin is superseded by the conscious reflection of personal sacrifice and the pragmatic necessities of blood donation. In violating the purity standards implemented by the government, the men in this study actively reiterate these civic ties, privileging the value of seeing like a citizen over the institutional tendencies of "seeing like a state."[54] The many faces of stranger-relationality embodied by these men accentuate the advantages of infrapolitics to resist state-authorized essentialism, the relationship those hidden transcripts share with public transgressions, and the narratives invigorated by these queer networks.

The statistical obsession of the sciences that undergird the donation process does little more than situate queer men as impure citizens. To resist these generalizations, queer men both pass and protest to disarticulate projections of affliction and stigma from their bodies. The hesitation of some men to continue donating blood may suggest that resistance has been thwarted. However, those who refrain from donation need not recite resistance in the same fashion to combat the deferral measures. Their initial infiltration of the system remains successful and their enduring discussions illustrate a continued engagement with the issue. More often than not, reproach to the state is dispersed through everyday transgressions that alter the consciousness of the people participating in the polis. Collective action is possible only after such transformations have manifested in the minds of social actors. The gaps between and among diverse actions are necessary for change. Social movements are like muscles—if you work the same angle consistently, they tend to plateau. Movements, like muscles, need the negative, the downtime, and an assortment of practices to grow and achieve strength.

The reciprocal forces of passing and protesting continue to be viable tactics of resistance against the logics of the blood ban. Each is a powerful device, but the two are most potent when in conversation with one another. The resistive potential of passing and protesting are not isolated to the deferral policy. In regards to issues like "don't ask, don't tell," for example, there are constant reminders in the public sphere that queers are serving in the military. Enlisted queers disrupt normative expectations of militarism, drawing attention to discourses of heterosexist exclusion. Passing and protesting are a corrective to this debilitating force, rousing possibilities for altering the consciousness of queer actors. When Americans are told the first U.S. soldier injured in Iraq is also gay, for instance, it draws attention to the number of queers serving in uniform. Those passing may not actively encourage such tabulations, but their very service gives space for exploring their presence. Conversely, those who have left the military (by force or by choice) and who elect to speak against government policies support those passing by propagating arguments for queers who cannot speak.

Where the true effect of these protests can be productively felt is in the stories that queer citizens carry back to their communities. Their experiences have the potential to influence local, and even federal, policies. While I want to avoid rendering hidden transcripts theoretically impotent by suggesting public discourses are needed to prove their effectiveness, there are emerging networks of resistance emanating from these practices. Again, dozens of protests against the blood ban are transpiring on high school, college, and university campuses every year. Along with "Fight to Give Life" there is now a student organization out of Harvard's Law School dedicated explicitly to combating these policies. Protests have been sparked at Stanford, the University of New Hampshire, the University of Vermont, the University of Arkansas, Bowling Green State University, and Dickinson College, among others.[55] These networks continue to take root in other settings as well. A sixteen-year-old high school student protesting at Jonathan Law High School in Connecticut told the *Advocate* she was speaking out because one queer student was excluded from the ritual.[56]

These networks of resistance remain imperative for dismantling the deferral policy. Certainly, the blood supply needs additional donors and queer men would provide countless amounts of liquid life. About thirty-eight thousand units of blood are required every day in the United States for transfusions alone and much more is required when factoring in blood products. Lifting the ban would alleviate blood deficits to a small degree, but the shortages have not been influential enough to initiate change. Losing current or potential donors, however, does spark anxiety for collection agencies. Calls by the ARC to relax the ban have not arisen solely from a desire to avoid charges of discrimination, but from the prospect of losing queer-friendly heterosexual donors early in life. The blood donation process, being articulated in the minds of those young citizens with prejudice and inequality, propagates unfavorable attitudes difficult to repair. The commitment to strangers generated by protests are not merely heartwarming for queers—they are essential. At the same time, the people most hurt by a scarcity of blood are not those masterminding these measures, but those occupying hospital beds. The possibilities for stranger-relationality are endless, but the system leaves few avenues for both resisting the guidelines and offering comfort to fellow citizens.

Although many people, including scores of queer men, express ambivalence toward the deferral policy, other donors continue to confront the questionnaire daily. In this light, the ban is ominous because of the false epistemological images of queer men it circulates. It is worth repeating that tens of thousands of people give blood every day. And every one of them confronts the question that asks: "are you a male who has had sexual contact with another male, even once, since 1977?" This question reinforces a model of citizenship that capitalizes on distrust and disconnectedness, not generosity and altruism among strangers. Until these measures are altered, queer men will continue to pass and protest, quietly building networks of resistance, constituting themselves as citizens outside the reach of repressive institutional discourses.

6

A Radical Tolerance of Experimentation

In the six years that unfolded between the BPAC meeting on blood donation in 2000 and the conference on deferral policies in 2006, a tidal wave of change enveloped the queer world. In June 2003 the United States Supreme Court made one of its most significant decisions of the year when it struck down sodomy laws that plagued gays and lesbians for decades. Months later, the highest judiciary court in Massachusetts ruled that same-sex relationships must be afforded a legal status that mirrors the privileges of heterosexual marriage. Not long after, the mayor of San Francisco defied state law by issuing marriage licenses to same-sex couples. As a response, President George Bush and factions on the right furthered their efforts to amend the Constitution to define marriage as being solely between a man and a woman in 2004. In a notoriously divisive move, the Episcopal Church ordained the first openly gay bishop in its history. LGBT culture was ever present on television shows ranging from *The Amazing Race, Will and Grace, Queer Eye for the Straight Guy, Survivor, Boy Meets Boy,* and *The L Word.*

In the midst of these events, the blood ban would periodically and with little fanfare creep its way into the news. Usually the spotlight would fall to students on a college or university campus who took issue with the measure, arguing that the deferrals violated antidiscrimination policies at their institution. One of these included a small college on the west coast that barely gained notice from the media. In May 2003 the student government of Southern Oregon University canceled their spring blood drive after a group of undergraduates complained that the deferrals stood in opposition to institutional protections for sexual orientation. In response to those objections, student officials requested that the American Red Cross not visit their campus. Amanda Guidero, a student government officer, told the gay and lesbian newsmagazine the *Advocate,* that "it took me four days to decide, and I can walk away knowing I made the right decision . . . I do believe those students had a legitimate concern."[1]

Always attempting to avoid public controversy, the Red Cross offered a typical middle-of-the-road statement about the decision. A public relations officer blandly noted that "you have to balance how much good you're doing with a safe blood supply with the bad feelings you're stirring in groups of people."[2] In this case, however, the "groups of people" described were not simply the unruly queer population often employed in state-sanctioned discourses—it was the governing branch of a student body. Here, the distorted public warning about a collection of people living in denial of the very dangers they pose to the polity fell on deaf ears. The "bad feelings" mentioned by the organization's representative were not simply those of the queer men being excluded, but those of a community reaffirming the bonds of social life among different kinds of people. And that difference was not feared, excluded, or dehumanized by the students at Southern Oregon University—it was valued.

Altering the contours of the blood ban is the focus of this concluding chapter. By advancing a rhetoric that prizes the desire for civic participation, the power of self-awareness over state-sanctioned monitoring, and the positive attributes of stranger-relationality, the ban can engender enriching forms of political praxis. Because the policy has been slow to evolve, citizens must continue formulating novel modes of resistance and advocate feasible alternatives to the current measure. Epistemological understandings of queer men rooted in false ontological categories present a perilous stubbornness to realizing communal transformation. While this book has expounded on many aspects of the exclusionary mandate, a final goal of this study is to augment the democratic potential for stimulating change. At its foundation, this project has sought to illuminate two underlying premises: the discursive power of the blood ban to stigmatize, denigrate, and ultimately marginalize queer men and the need to formulate innovative civic actions to reconstitute these defaming effects.

Primarily, *Banning Queer Blood* has magnified the material consequences generated by convoluted institutional rhetorics stemming from a matrix that includes the state, the law, science, and the media. These duplicitous discourses intersect at various points in the public sphere, fabricating and facilitating injurious caricatures that do violence to queer lives. Repeatedly, men who have sex with men are couched in a language of disease, contagion, and danger. The imagined queer man is one who is unaware of his diseased body, yet acting with maximum consciousness to the detriment of the polity. This paradigm of social denial envisions queer men as knowing, but refusing to acknowledge, that they are more susceptible to contracting and transmitting HIV/AIDS than their heterosexual counterparts. Queer men, from this perspective, always subvert the productive possibilities of the blood donation ritual.

No regard is ever given to their roles as conscientious donors or citizens acting from an ethic of care.

In spite of troublesome dynamics manifest in transcripts of official proceedings within the health establishment, the infrapolitics associated with the blood ban offers insight into the cultural practices that resist discriminatory policies. The final element of this study, therefore, incorporated the voices of men who have either lied to donate blood or protested the guidelines and thus refused to conceal their sexuality. While resistance by passing and protesting are often seen as separate forms of opposition, they are two sides of the same coin, existing dialogically to resist the blood ban. We need not romanticize the actions of these men to comprehend the significance of their opposition. These donors reclaim their personal experiences, narrating their life stories and regulating their bodies outside the reach of the powerful. They insert their bodies into the ritual space and call into question the epidemiological knowledge propagated by blood agencies. They move beyond narrowly constructed conceptions of citizenship resting on the language of civil rights, providing a catalyst for imagining inclusive appeals outside the constraining dictums of "tolerance."[3]

The blanket discrimination confronting queer men is alarming for all people desiring a more robust democracy that values both the well-being of the polity and the blood supply. Without proper justification, a small number of women and men are permitted to isolate several well-intentioned and healthy citizens. It is time to stop constructing these donors as a disruptive force that threatens the polity and to begin treating them as a source of strengthening social bonds among strangers. To accomplish this, discourses of rationality that insinuate themselves as self-evident and civically prudent must continue to be challenged. Although queer donors clearly identify differences among themselves, they are persistently essentialized by institutional actors who knowingly disregard pertinent information that would ease public stigma and instigate communal identifications. This stigmatization is hazardous for democratic culture, undermining the salutary political potential inherent in difference and reifying a fictitious common sense about identity, health, and civic participation.

CORRESPONDING RISKS

Despite my criticisms of the medical and scientific community, I am sympathetic to arguments concerning the fundamental import of blood. At no time do I dispute that blood is an essential element for sustaining life, helping thousands of people to live longer and more freely each year. But the fact that blood is a basic necessity does not negate that agencies such as the FDA should be scrutinized, their practices refuted, and their meetings boycotted. Vigorous democratic practice sometimes necessitates uncomfortable challenges to normativities. Indeed, the more sacred a practice the more important the need to rouse criticism that resists taken-for-granted judgments that marginalize citizens. As uncomfortable and unsettling as it may seem, protesting and boycotting blood drives may be the most effective retort to the policies. Knowing the frequency with which people in this country need blood, I was shy to advocate such measures until I became acutely aware of how mean-spirited the policies were, at least in their consequences if not also in their intent. Boycotting may not be the only method to capturing the attention of the FDA, but it is certainly the most effective. Even among agencies that now support relaxing the ban, there is a continued return to a rhetoric that is hostile to queer men. Take, for example, this extended exchange I had with the ARC while attempting to gather information about the legal implications of the blood ban. The letter is problematic in both its content and its form, but offers insight into how the ban is sustained. In an e-mail to the organization, I wrote:

> Hello there. I'm writing about blood donation and was hoping to talk to a representative about some of the legal aspects of donor deferrals (specifically gay men). Accuracy is very important to me and if your offices could point me in the direction of an appropriate contact that would be much appreciated.
>
> Thanks in advance for your help,
> Jeff

In return, I received an almost immediate response from "Blood," with the following lengthy message:

> Dear Mr. Bennett:
>
> Thank you for contacting the American Red Cross. Certainly discrimination—automatic judgement based on untrue or irrelevant facts—is unacceptable.[4] The American Red Cross makes all of its services available to anyone in need with no regard for age, race, lifestyle, ability to pay or any other qualification.
>
> The safety of the blood supply is the top priority of the American Red Cross. The Red Cross follows all Food and Drug Administration (FDA) (www.fda.gov) guidelines to protect the safety of the blood supply, including the current deferral of men who have had sex with other men (MSM) even once since 1977.

Some worst-case estimates by the Centers for Disease Control (CDC) conducted in 2000 suggest modifying the MSM criterion to a five-year period may allow an additional 1,200 units of HIV-positive blood to enter the system for testing each year (based on CDC-estimated HIV prevalence rate of 2 percent in this population).

This is a public health issue, not a social policy issue. The American Red Cross cannot change its procedures in a way that would result in increased numbers of infectious donations in our blood supply.

If the Public Health Service could assure the American Red Cross that introducing previously deferred donors into the donor pool could be accommodated without increasing risk, we would support appropriate actions to do so.

The reason that testing alone is not sufficient is because of a phenomenon called "the window period." The "window period" is defined as the time frame between when an individual has been infected with a virus and when the virus can be detected by blood tests. Depending on which tests are used, the window period may be as long as 45 days. Because individuals who are engaged in high-risk behavior may be in the "window period" of infection (but are under the impression that they are "negative") we ask these individuals to refrain from blood donation to ensure the safest possible blood supply for patients.

Excluding high-risk individuals from blood donation is not a comment on the donor's judgement, behavior, morals or lifestyle in any way. Rather, the intent is very straightforward: Where we know that a specific behavior or characteristic creates an increased risk of carrying a dangerous transmissible virus—whatever that behavior or characteristic might be—such persons must not donate blood in order to protect vulnerable transfusion recipients. Based on other FDA regulations and guidelines, the Red Cross and other blood centers apply this approach to many behaviors and characteristics in addition to male-to-male sex.

We hope this clarification is helpful. Thank you for sharing your concerns.

Sincerely,
Biomedical Inquiry
The Public Inquiry Center
American Red Cross

I share this exchange because it exhibits in a single page many of the problems spawned by the deferral measure. This correspondence reflects the mentality of those who have incorporated troubling and questionable information as a matter of common sense. Based on its detailed and nonresponsive execution, there is reason to believe this is a standard reply sent to people who question the policy. It advances several claims typical in the blood-ban debate and then loosely supports them with evidence. While the person composing this message was obviously well versed in the rhetoric espoused by the FDA, he or she missed several important points.

First and foremost, my inquiry was never answered. At no point was the "legal" element of my question addressed. Rather, the response resituates the reader to view the issue through the lens of science, with the Public Health Service and the FDA as the final authorities on the matter. However, there is no resolution to the legal aspects of the ban that supposedly sustain their "safeguards." To be certain, my many attempts over the years to secure clarifying information from the ARC and the FDA about the legalities of the deferral policy have been passed over. Although the ARC's Office of General Counsel was supposed to clarify the legal ramifications, my queries have consistently fallen on deaf ears. Even questions about the collection of deferred donor names, and their subsequent entry into a database system that is kept by the ARC, have been met with silence.

Aside from the overt dismissal of the question, problematic features of this message accentuate the mentality of those who imagine queer men as diseased. It is intriguing that the ARC defines how the term "discrimination" should be understood. Recall that the writer classified "discrimination" as "*automatic* judgement based on untrue or irrelevant facts" (my emphasis). It would seem then that the systematic exclusion of queer men is not in fact discrimination because it is deliberately contemplated and intentionally conceived. Of course, slavery, genocide, war, and a number of other atrocities used as overt tools of discrimination would also seem to lie outside the boundaries of this definition because they are based on "rational" deliberation and evidence that is "true" and "relevant." The extent to which methodological *process* is highlighted needs to be underscored. The elusive and spontaneous nature of queer sexuality is constructed as the antithesis to rational deliberation, inciting only impoverishment to the blood supply. Disease is made wholly present and the responsibilities of the donor and communal altruism are eclipsed. Further, a number of people sitting on the BPAC have clearly stated that the window period is not a significant issue. Scientific testing measures are almost universally safe, as evidenced by the lack of infected blood penetrating the system.[5]

Further, the allusion to unprotected anal sex is ubiquitous in this message. Notice the strategic ambiguity that is prevalent in the text. The representative wrote: "Rather, the intent is very straightforward: Where we know that a specific behavior or characteristic creates an increased risk of carrying a dangerous transmissible virus—whatever that behavior or characteristic might be—such persons must not donate blood in order to protect vulnerable transfusion recipients." While there is an indication of a "specific behavior," the sexual act is one that the ARC will not name. They are content to leave the reader guessing when they assert "whatever that behavior or characteristic may be." Despite the vague language, there is no pluralized term in this thin description of sex, no indication that multiple forms of sexuality and sexual behavior exist. Men who have sex with men are again reduced, by implication, to anal sex, but that very act is always veiled.

This ruinous line of reasoning is supported in part by the organization of the message that foregrounds disease and then moves into the sexual relations between queer men. Like the meetings held by the BPAC, the text deploys cultural stereotypes about queer men to further a specific agenda. It presumes familiar negative associations on the part of the audience in order to advance ill-conceived generalizations and then uses those unwarranted associations to forward unfounded claims. The image of the queer donor preying on helpless transfusion victims is introduced once more to undermine the extent to which queer men are enabled to be full citizen actors.

UNDOING IMPURITY

Throughout this project I have been careful to recognize that science and medicine have, in many ways, had a positive impact on the lives of tens of thousands, even millions, of people living with HIV and AIDS. I do not question that countless people have benefited from advancements in drug research and studies that delimit the nature of the agents that cause disease and instigate the degeneration of the body. However, it is equally important to recognize the extent to which these hard-won changes have been brought about by citizens who questioned the system, demanding that people stop dying because of institutional neglect and corporate greed. With that history in mind, this final segment considers how we can begin undoing impurity, moving away from official discourses that imagine queer men as contagions and toward a civic project that emphasizes the productive nature of their citizenship. Rather than assert any particular model as the correct one for conceptualizing cultural practices, it is best to approach such matters in a Foucauldian manner, advocating polymorphous forms of actions and recognizing that some exploits will be successful and others will not.

Scores of theorists and activists have argued that power must be reiterated to hold its place in people's everyday lives, as power's discursive formations do not exist statically or without change.[6] Power reproduces itself not in a linear fashion or "from above," but through the interworkings of the quotidian. Power is not something to escape, but something to confront, because "relations of power are not essentially contested; they are contingently contested."[7] In short, the specifics of a situation offer the tools for generating tactics of resistance against oppressive regimes. The blood ban universalizes MSM rather than consider the radical recontextualization provided by individual bodies. As such, queer donors must persistently stress the differences among themselves to oppose the ontological positioning of science and the law. Asserting the uniqueness of one's sense of citizenship will not always subvert normative harms, and can even potentially repeat the discourses it seeks to displace, but such iterations are one starting point for articulating new illocutions of identity. In no way is this attempting to signal that queer men should stigmatize one another (or people of other orientations) based on their sexual practices. Rather, queer men need to recognize how their identities are being used to mark them as embodiments of disease and innovatively counter that stigma. In doing so, I hope that resisting the blood ban will contribute to, in Kenneth Plummer's words, a "delight of difference."[8] Rather than constrain difference to a mere fear of the "other," diverse identifications could be seen as a productive mechanism in cultivating volunteers. Critics such as Jeffrey Weeks have recognized this potential, advocating for a "radical tolerance of experimentation" to enhance public culture.[9]

The metaphor of "experimentation" here is intentionally selected to run contrary to the scientific medical standards embraced by the FDA. The word "experimentation" connotes laboratories of creativity to affect social change, not static ontologies that deplete the vigor of civic life. For Weeks, citizens should operate these experiments with a doctrine of three basic beliefs: the principles of "refusal," "curiosity," and "innovation."[10] These three intertwined places of argument are heuristics for structuring modes of agonistic confrontation. The ubiquitous nature of the blood ban's diabolical discourses in the public sphere requires multiple reproach and these touchtones are productive starting points for dissolving these social barriers.

"Refusal" suggests that we question anything deemed self-evident. While seemingly simple, calling into question sacred practices such as blood donation and ideological scripts underwritten by science can be enormously challenging. But by asserting such efforts, citizens can move beyond the normalizing tendencies in the practices of everyday life. Importantly, this is not meant to be a suspension of all beliefs, where actors position themselves as objective observers of the social body. Rather, it promotes an interrogation of those norms and practices that are taken for granted, even when they exist to the detriment of others. In the rhetoric of the blood ban, for example, citizens of all sexual orientations might recognize the devastating effects that normalization, and hence stigmatization, have on public culture. By exploring the essentializing tendencies of agencies such as the FDA, citizens enable themselves to scrutinize the discursive production of some bodies as negligible and others safe from contagion. In particular, citizens should refuse the supposedly objective frames of science and the alleged transparency of "risk."

For all of its benefits and necessities, science and medicine are rhetorics imbued with cultural values. These rhetorics must be challenged, questioned, and engaged. It takes little research to find compelling examples of how cultural values constitute and couch the processes, judgments, and conclusions of science and medicine. For example, for decades schoolchildren were taught a standard curriculum for reproduction that lives on today. Children in sex education are told that reproduction begins with the man's sperm and the woman's egg. According to the narrative, thousands of sperm are released from the male body and each of them competes to penetrate the egg. In this tale, the sperm are competitors and it is the fastest, strongest sperm that will reach the egg and pierce its walls. The egg, it would seem, remains docile, waiting for something to happen. Today, feminism has taught us that this narrative is rife with male and female stereotypes. The male sperm are imagined as competitive and must be sturdy and quick. The egg is seemingly without agency and at the mercy of the sperm. Further research about reproduction, inflected by the contributions of feminism and changes in attitudes toward gender, has since argued that the egg plays an integral role in determining which sperm is permitted to take part in fertilization. The constitutive features of culture offering form to these narratives are central to interpreting the facts being presented. Such discourses are a ubiquitous part of the scientific process and hard work is required to undo the naturalization of information perpetuated as fact.[11]

When the ARC contended the blood ban was a "public health" issue, it attempted to invoke the credibility of science. In their eyes it was not a "social policy," meaning the measure does not carry the connotation of subjectivity and emotion typically divorced from normative perceptions of science. In the debate surrounding the blood ban, this guise of objectivity is central to the policy's sturdiness. Government agents are able to elide the contributions of queer men by positioning their sexual practices as objectively impure, not subjectively diversified. One official at the FDA, for instance, asserted that "there are legitimate concerns about stigmatizing, and it certainly makes individuals feel as if something were wrong with them, and that's not OK—but for the greater good, we've tried to err on being overly cautious."[12] There is in this discourse full recognition that discrimination is not only transpiring, but having a negative effect in the community where it is being executed. Nonetheless, "caution" implies "risk," and "greater good" offers an excuse for dismissing claims to full civic participation. The constructs of "risk" and "caution" evolve in a deliberative setting, but the forums consistently suggest a binary that squarely positions queer men as unsafe, unruly, and by extension impure. Such rhetoric is reminiscent of Hannah Arendt's conclusion that the nation-state claims "to be above all classes, completely independent of society and its particular interests, the true and only representative of the nation as a whole."[13] The very health of the public rests on the isolation of queer men.

It is striking to note that the ban was not revisited in the years 1997 and 2000 because policy makers wanted to alleviate social stigma. Rather, officials believed that expanding the donor pool might help the dwindling national blood supply. The need for blood is increasing by 1 percent each year, and donations are declining at the same rate. Couple this finding with demographic shifts, "an aging population that uses more blood while donating less," and the exigency of cultivating fresh blood dramatically increases.[14] More recently it was discovered that the number of eligible donors was significantly lower than had been projected. A study released in 2007 found there are about sixty-seven million fewer donors than typically estimated.[15] Although some people have argued that lifting the ban will not sizably increase donations, the proceedings of the BPAC indicated that they would never really know how many queer men might contribute until the policy was relaxed.

Knowing that a moratorium on the ban might not significantly increase donations could appear problematic for opponents of the blood ban. But this is a shortsighted understanding of cost. Advocates of repealing the ban must instigate arguments that refuse traditional cost-benefit analysis. Again, this project does not claim to have all of the answers to this vexing problem. But there is little denying that there are other forms of "cost" in this debate that need voice. Young donors could be lost forever because of perceived discrimination. This is an unmistakable cost. A questionnaire that tells heterosexuals they are immune from disease and that queer people are inherently dirty is a cost. Telling young queers their sexuality is so hazardous that no precaution can curtail the risk of HIV comes at a cost. The idea of cost extends far beyond the number of new donors that can be attracted, whatever that number might be.

The refusal of taken-for-granted normativities is part and parcel of Weeks's conception of "curiosity." Under the rubric of curiosity, citizens engage in critiques of those things that appear most self-evident to explore the potential that lies outside the narrow casting of dominant discourses. It must be acknowledged that all people are susceptible to disease and that the struggle against HIV/AIDS is something to be shared, not used as a site of discrimination that further alienates people from their communities. Curiosity offers the opportunity to rethink long-held generalizations of queer men. Let there be little doubt—not everyone will universally subscribe to these notions. If one were to take a sample of people who had to undergo a blood transfusion and were asked if they wanted to receive the blood of a heterosexual or a queer man, the latter may lose out. But forcing questions about *why* one would want a specific kind of blood and the cultural norms that accompany such thinking would prove pedagogically and democratically valuable. A curious predisposition to democratic culture would have us not only reform the questionnaires, but would also further efforts to educate publics about the ban and reformulate arguments stressing "civil rights."

The FDA should take the appropriate steps to reword questionnaires so that specific sexual behaviors are taken into account. Inquiring about sexual practices, safe sex, and relational monogamy for all donors is the most effective way to ensure the safety of the blood supply and increase donations. Employing a deductive set of inquires, the forms could begin with the number of sex partners a donor of any sexuality has had since the last time they gave blood and progress from that point. If a person acknowledges multiple partners, a few simple questions about precaution and risk-taking could help to determine donor eligibility. Blood collection agencies have an interest in asking donors about sexual history, and grown adults should be able to answer these questions frankly. With the addition of a couple of questions, the FDA could reposition the forms to be grounded in educational motives and not based on heterosexism. To boot, all traditional testing measures would remain in place.

While I recognize collection agencies do not wish to meddle in people's private affairs, they already do so with the present deferral question. When organizations claim they do not want to be intrusive, it is important to recognize with whom they do not wish to be invasive. Uncounted numbers of queer men have been deferred because of menacing probes. When agencies argue that they are distancing themselves from asking about specific sexual practices to avoid embarrassing people, they are talking exclusively about heterosexual donors. Queer men who practice safe sex should be sought after more aggressively than straight people who do not.

Expanding the scope of the questionnaire could help educate the public about risky sexual practices such as unprotected vaginal or anal sex. Agencies might also provide educational materials for citizens, encouraging them to get tested for communicable diseases, indicating where such testing is done, and specifying how those tests are performed. If blood collection agencies do not wish to support such activities because they fear attracting populations that could put the blood supply at risk, they might at least point people toward organizations that can provide information about safe sex and methods for avoiding STDs. Currently, the system does little more than determine that individuals do not qualify for donation and then dismisses them.

Additionally, LGBT lobby groups must offer more attention to the ban if it is to be overturned in the near future. Marriage-obsessed organizations such as the Human Rights Campaign, for example, occasionally release a statement to the press when the BPAC meets. Beyond that, there are few organized attempts to abolish the discriminatory question that ritually excludes queer men in places of civic import. To be certain, the sensitive nature of the subject may make it difficult for groups to garner public support to reproach the government. Issues such as marriage are in many ways easier to debate in institutional settings because of the emphasis on individual rights and secular economic arguments.

One result of this absence is that many people, of all sexual orientations, are unaware that the ban exists. During the time this manuscript was being composed, people would look at me with wonder and amazement that such highly problematic and discriminatory policies subsist. Professors, healthcare workers, students, relatives—all were nonplussed by the rationale guiding the FDA. A friend of mine in Manhattan, Kansas, conveyed that a Red Cross volunteer in her graduate seminar in Gender and Communication insisted that the ban was not active. A gay male acquaintance called me after I sent out solicitations for interviews and noted that he had no idea the ban was in place. A close friend who directed a competitive speech program in the Midwest encouraged a student to use the blood ban as an oratory topic. Both were shocked when they received critiques from an "out" gay judge who insisted that the student must be mistaken. Because these policies are so infrequently discussed, the ritual continually catches queer men off guard when they attempt to donate blood.

Further, activists need to move away from an emphasis on "civil rights" when combating the deferral policy. Although such arguments have proven effective at pushing forward marriage, adoption, and employment rights, these appeals do little more than offer proponents of the blood ban a formula for victory. When the LGBT community attaches itself to arguments that revolve around *rights* and *tolerance* rather than *responsibility* and *inclusion* it invites almost immediate dismissal. During a meeting of the BPAC, for example, one member exclaimed, "I don't think that people, necessarily, have a right to be a blood donor."[16] And right he is. There is no constitutional or statutory provision that secures giving blood as essential to life, liberty, and the pursuit of happiness.

Queer theorists such as Lisa Duggan and Michael Warner have justifiably remained skeptical about the results of a rights-based model of activism.[17] Often, identifications based on "civil rights" conform to a normative discourse that attempts to disable queer populations from engaging in democratic participation on their own terms. These accepted frames, that often subtly stress assimilation, do not merely suggest a form of passivity, but the very terms of the relationship being constituted. Such conceptions are problematic for queer citizens who likely foster varying experiences, opportunities, and restrictions from their heterosexual counterparts. When read against the powerful ritual of blood donation, it is important to question if lifting the restrictions would valorize the positive effects difference can have on the polity or simply resituate queers in heterosexual hegemony.

The students of Southern Oregon University offer an appealing alternative. Simply because donation is not a "civil right" does not mean the policies are not discriminatory. Perhaps it is not a matter of pushing the government and the blood industry for donation privileges. Rather, it might be a matter of pushing the agencies away all together. If direct appeals to the FDA are decisively ineffective, then protesting and boycotting blood drives is the next logical step to securing reasonable policies. As citizens increasingly resist the measures at the local level, pressure will be put on blood agencies to lean more heavily on the FDA. Concerns raised by the ARC about the numbers of young donors who are opting out of the giving process because of perceived discrimination indicate such cultural politics are working and furthering these tactics of dissent could be productive for people desiring change.

Along with refusal and curiosity, Weeks encourages "innovation" in order "to seek out in our reflection those things that have never been thought or imagined."[18] One of the more interesting findings of this study came from the chapter on passing and protesting. Queer men were transforming themselves into civic actors, even at the expense of revealing their sexual practices. While these men should not have to discipline their citizenship to accommodate their desires, it is telling that they are in fact willing to make sacrifices in order to give blood and help transform the polity. In this way, democratic practice, indeed power itself, is coming from below. Contrary to the antediluvian beliefs of agencies such as the FDA, these men offer new ways of conceptualizing citizenship for all people precisely because they embody multiple sacrifices (both their identity and their blood). They subtly reorganize structures of power to affect change in their community by recognizing the limits of demonizing difference.

The actions of these men offer the opportunity to rethink how difference is conceptualized in the polity. These donors sustain and supplement notions of what Iris Marion Young has called "communicative democracy." They lend to the creation of positive associations with difference that require "a plurality of perspectives, speaking styles, and ways of expressing the particularity of social situation as well as the general applicability of principles."[19] More important still, these men disrupt the traditional workings of the polis. They force questions about the most basic norms of culture—those involving health, community, citizenship, and diversity. They challenge generalizations about the dangers they supposedly present, innovatively reconceptualizing their position from abject other to empowered citizen. Far from utopian visions of unity, these deferred donors spark the kinds of discussions that keep our culture productively invigorated.

On a basic level, then, queer activists and their allies must innovatively protest the harms instigated by the blood ban. Such efforts are easy enough to initiate locally, as evidenced by student protests held on dozens of college campuses annually. As mentioned in the previous chapter, a student group called "Fight to Give Life" staged a national protest in the spring of 2006, infiltrating blood centers across the country. The students presented letters to the volunteers, hoping their concerns would be passed along to those at the top of agency bureaucracies. Harvard Law's student group "Blood Sense" has one of the most forward thinking plans for altering the ban and displays both the problems with the ban and possible solutions on their web site.[20] Students and faculty at Sonoma State University and San Jose State University (SJSU) in California were featured on NPR because of their efforts to overturn the ban.[21] These are not simply LGBT activists, but young citizens taking control of the future direction of their community.[22]

The efforts of students at places such as Sonoma State and SJSU have not fallen on deaf ears. Their representative is one of the few members of Congress who, at the time of this writing, has publicly questioned the FDA's stance. U.S. representative Sam Farr was alerted to the measure not by queer organizers, but by a Santa Cruz high school student who had concerns about the policy.[23] During a House Appropriations Committee hearing in April 2008, Farr grilled the FDA about not revisiting the policy in the face of new technology. Farr was questioning Dr. Jesse Goodman, the director for Biologics Evaluation and Research at the FDA. Goodman insisted that gay men held too great a risk for HIV and Hepatitis to be donors. In what was supposed to be a statistical shocker, Goodman asserted that queer men have an "800-fold increase in HIV compared to first-time blood donors, and a 1,000-fold increase in HIV compared to repeat blood donors." Note the ways queer men and other citizens are constructed in this sentence. Heterosexuals are offered the qualifiers of "donors" and "repeat donors." Rather than contemplate if queer donors would harbor similar safety records, queer men are left on the level of disease—that's *all* they are in this equation. The nobility of heterosexual blood donors is underscored by their lack of diseases, and by extension their lack of unseemly sex. But again, regardless of their relational monogamy, safe-sex practices, or consciousness about their HIV-status, queer men are always already contagious.

There are a variety of innovative measures for launching campaigns against the blood ban. The Internet, for example, has proven to be a valuable medium for the LGBT movement to raise consciousness about controversial issues. Dr. Laura Schlessinger's disturbing remarks that gays and lesbians were a mistake of nature, for instance, were addressed almost entirely over the Internet. It was not a barrage of protestors that eventually led to the cancellation of Dr. Laura's show. Instead, it was the result of four people who developed the web site "stopdrlaura.com." The site received 14 million hits in the first two months it was made public. Advertisers took note and the program was deemed too risky for sponsors.

When discussing the merits of queer men as blood donors, activists would be wise to stress a model that highlights the variability of the queer community and the similarities shared by blood donors of all sexual orientations. Time and again throughout this rhetoric there is little data presented about the kinds of people who tend to donate blood. There is almost no understanding of the queer men who would give blood. This information is lacking in large part because neither the ARC nor the FDA will relax the ban to study donor rates. As suggested by the testimony of the men in chapter 5, however, it may be that donors who wish to give usually do so for altruistic reasons. Far from presenting a danger to the polity, these men have much to contribute to the well-being of the communities in which they live. Repeat donors tend to be especially health conscious, but it is difficult to ascertain the extent to which these patterns exist in the queer community.

BLOOD WORK

Despite shortages, it is doubtful that the prohibition on queer blood will be fully revoked in the near future. With changing political tides and gay rights advances, however, such exclusions will likely erode into prejudices of the past. If anything, in the near future it is more probable that the deferral period will be dropped to five years, or perhaps to one. Policy, especially in regard to health, tends to evolve slowly over time to offer the illusion of carefully thought-out deliberation when other motivations such as public backlash and litigation are often at the heart of the matter. Although some might be tempted to claim a five-year deferral is a sign of "progress," we should be wary of such proclamations. The same logic that reifies disease for the current ban would also inspire the five-year or one-year rule. There would remain a double standard between queer citizens and their heterosexual counterparts, with a continued neglect of responsibility, altruism, and community. Nonetheless, in the year 2000 the ban was upheld by a single vote on the BPAC. Several members wanted to relax it in an attempt to incorporate more donors. But altering these regulations has proven to be a tediously slow process. Initial amendments to the policy are likely to be minimal, even with the plethora of evidence illustrating the FDA's decision to be misguided. This includes appeals from the ARC, the American Association of Blood Banks, and America's Blood Centers to overhaul the policy.

Regardless of the tactics deployed by queer activists and their allies, more pronounced efforts at directly challenging blood policies must transpire. The students at Southern Oregon University did little more than ask the ARC not to visit campus for the spring blood drive because it violated the school's antidiscrimination policies. While this isolated incident garnered little publicity, a large number of protests might generate needed discussions. The shyness of the ARC to field negative publicity might force the issue in enough locations that a serious reconsideration of the ban will be required. Changes will happen only when communities take the steps to embrace the value of difference in their polity and the benefits to be reaped from recognizing diversity and inclusion. Agonism, as Chantal Mouffe has argued, is required for the development and preservation of a healthy and pluralistic democratic culture and polity.[24]

During the past two decades there has been a silencing of dissent by people who oppose the blood ban. The benevolent nature of giving blood, and the human necessity for receiving it under precarious circumstances, assuredly makes protest more difficult to conceptualize in the face of the positive work collection agencies do. However, as the world comes to accept that we are all equal, it is imperative to underscore that we are not. The queer community has much to offer the larger polity, including those in need of blood. Rather than compromise their bodies and abilities, queer men and their allies must continue stressing the benefits of difference and the power of their diversity.

Notes

CHAPTER 1

1. John F. Harris, "God Gave U.S. 'What We Deserve' Falwell Says," *Washington Post,* September 14, 2001.

2. See William F. Buckley, "Invoking God's Thunder," *The National Review Online,* September 18, 2001; Katha Pollitt, "Put Out No Flags," *The Nation,* October 8, 2001, 9.

3. American Red Cross, "September 11," 17.

4. The word "queer" will be the preferred term of this book. Because the FDA bans "men who have sex with other men" from giving blood, it is not always appropriate to use the word "gay" to describe donors. Privileging this term is not without its complications. While the medical community highlights behavior over identity, organizations opposing the ban tend to identify as "gay." Nonetheless, the prison house of language dictates the need for words and "queer" seems most appropriate. Some exceptions to this rule will be the use of the word "gay" in historical references where "queer" is not as contextually appropriate and the self-identifications of men in chapter 5.

5. Bayer, "Blood and AIDS," 25.

6. Please see the Red Cross homepage at www.redcross.org. The emphasis is mine.

7. The letter sent to me by the Red Cross in the last chapter of this book highlights such discourse. Or, visit the Red Cross homepage at www.redcross.org.

8. Young, "Abjection and Oppression," 209.

9. All men and women are informed to think of themselves in relation to the men who have sex with men. Men are asked directly about their sexual lives in relation to other men. Women, conversely, are asked if they have had sex with a man who has had sex with another man in the past year. In both cases it is the impurity of queer men that marks and rhetorically pollutes other bodies.

10. It should be said at the outset of this book that women who have sex with women are allowed to donate blood. In this sense, it could be suggested that the policy is not hostile to queer bodies, or that the policy is neither heterosexist nor homophobic because some queers are incorporated in the donor pool. However, as this text will argue, the exclusion of any group based on chronic stereotypes, state monitoring of the body, the use of science to control those bodies, and the false construction of

"bad blood" have consequences that stretch far beyond the lives of only men who have sex with men. The maliciousness of the deferral policy has disturbing implication for larger notions of purity, kinship, choice, and community, which in turn has ramifications for struggles in other realms of public life.

11. Scott, *Domination and the Arts of Resistance,* 2.

12. Ibid., 55.

13. Like Foucault, Scott recognizes that power is never wholly discreet and such practices never travel a straight line. Ibid., 5.

14. For an extended discussion of "tactics," see de Certeau, *Practice of Everyday Life,* 29–42.

15. U.S. Army Medical Service, *Blood Program in World War II,* xiii.

16. There is evidence to support the argument that Germans may have taken blood from people in concentration camps, though it is difficult to know if they were able to transport it to troops. Gisella Perl writes, "The sight which greeted us when we entered Bloc VII is one never to be forgotten. From the cages along the walls about six hundred panic-stricken, trembling young women were looking at us with silent pleading in their eyes. The other hundred were lying on the ground, pale, faint, bleeding. Their pulse was almost inaudible, their breathing strained and deep rivers of blood were flowing around their bodies. Big, strong S.S. men were going from one to the other sticking tremendous needles into their veins and robbing their undernourished, emaciated bodies of their last drop of blood. The German army needed blood plasma! *Rassenschande* or contamination with 'inferior Jewish blood' was forgotten. We were too 'inferior' to live, but not too inferior to keep the German army alive with our blood. Besides, nobody would know. The blood donors, along with the other prisoners of Auschwitz would never live to tell their tale." *I Was a Doctor in Auschwitz,* 74–75.

17. Bordo, "The Body and the Production of Femininity," 13.

18. Butler, "Imitation and Gender Insubordination," 27.

19. Bell, *Ritual Theory,* 220.

20. Ibid., 204.

21. Lister, *Citizenship,* 3.

22. Pocock, "The Ideal of Citizenship," 37.

23. Althusser, *Politics and History,* 62.

24. Butler, *Psychic Life of Power,* 10–11.

25. Lister, *Citizenship,* 3.

26. Miller, *Cultural Citizenship,* 39.

27. Joseph Carens gives particular emphasis to the notion of context, recognizing that moral judgments, themselves complex configurations, are further abstracted by theoretical considerations. See *Culture, Citizenship, and Community,* 4.

28. Kymlicka, *Multicultural Citizenship,* 125.

29. I first encountered these regulations in Miller, *Cultural Citizenship,* 53. See the U.S. Citizenship and Immigration Services website for naturalization requirements: http://www.uscis.gov.

30. Ibid.

31. For an excellent account of the development of blood-donor pools, see Starr, *Blood*.

32. Ibid., xi.

33. Ibid., x.

34. Ibid., 350.

35. Of course, this depends on the blood product being collected. While people are not usually paid for whole blood, they can be paid for donating plasma.

36. Starr, *Blood,* 186–197.

37. Titmuss's assertion that only 10 percent of all blood came from donors has been refuted by a number of authors. See Murray, "Poisoned Gift," and Starr, *Blood.*

38. Some scholars take exception to the idea there was a surplus of nonvoluntary donors in the American blood system. See Starr, *Blood,* 240. Also, Murray, "Poisoned Gift."

39. These quotations are sent out by the Red Cross national office and are posted on a variety of web pages. See, for example, the Leigh Valley homepage in Pennsylvania at http://www.redcrosslv.org/blood/faq.html and the Chicago Red Cross homepage at http://www.chicagoredcross.org/giveblood/bloodfaqs.htm.

40. Pieplow, "AIDS, Blood Banks and the Court," 617.

41. Ibid., 613.

42. Starr, *Blood,* 268.

43. To be sure, the United States was not the only country that grappled with a national struggle over the contamination of their blood supply. Japan, for example, had long prided itself for its national purity. AIDS was considered little more than an American disease. Ibid., 283.

44. Bayer, "Blood and AIDS," 23.

45. Jonathan Adler, "Bloodless," *Advocate (on-line edition),* November 21, 2005.

46. Institute of Medicine, *HIV and the Blood Supply,* 285.

47. In the early days of the crisis, some officials at the White House attempted to draft legislation making it a crime for gay men to donate blood. See Shilts, *And the Band Played On,* 295; hereafter cited as *Band.*

48. Hochberg, "HIV/AIDS and Blood Donation Policies," 250.

49. Importantly, there are several groups of people who cannot give. Having lived or visited particular parts of the world (such as England or portions of Africa) provides supposedly sufficient cause to reject some people's blood.

50. Institute of Medicine, *HIV and the Blood Supply,* 112.

51. Asen and Brouwer, *Counterpublics and the State,* 9.

52. Triechler, *How to Have Theory in an Epidemic,* 18.

53. Ibid., 76.

54. See Young, *Intersecting Voices.* Also, Warner, *Publics and Counterpublics;* Berlant and Warner, "Sex in Public"; Pezzullo, "Resisting 'National Breast Cancer Awareness Month'"; Fraser, *Justice Interruptus.*

55. See Crimp, *AIDS: Cultural Analysis.*

56. Patton, *Globalizing AIDS,* 50.

57. Yingling, *AIDS and the National Body.*

58. Foucault, *History of Sexuality,* 118.

59. Duster, *Backdoor to Eugenics,* 131.

60. Condit and Lucaites, *Crafting Equality,* xii–xiii.

61. Vaid, *Virtual Equality,* 106.

62. Ewick and Silbey, *Common Place of Law,* 232.

63. Darsey, *Prophetic Tradition and Radical Rhetoric,* 184.

64. BPAC, *57th Meeting,* 184.

65. Bayer, "Blood and AIDS"; Institute of Medicine, *HIV and the Blood Supply.*

66. Of course, such broad symptomatic guesses raise problems. Shilts, *Band,* 238.

67. Starr, *Blood,* 272.

68. Ibid., 293.

69. See, for example, Piliavin and Callero, *Giving Blood,* 240.

70. Shilts, *Band,* 309.

71. Kelly, "Liability of Blood Banks," 466.

72. Starr, *Blood,* 317.

73. Bayer, "Blood and AIDS," 25.

74. It has been widely posited that the AIDS crisis in many ways solidified the movement in important political and cultural ways.

75. Importantly, 2000 was the last time the issue was publicly revisited. Since George W. Bush took office scientists at national science organizations have had difficulty including sexuality in the most mundane of studies. Projects that included the words "men who have sex with other men" had a laborious time attracting federal funding. It is not surprising that the issue of blood donation has not seen daylight since. See Erica Goode, "Certain Words Can Trip Up AIDS Grants, Scientists Say," *New York Times,* April 18, 2003, A10; Nicholas Kristof, "No Time to Get Squeamish," *New York Times,* May 9, 2003, A31; Bob Herbert, "The Big Chill at the Lab," *New York Times,* November 3, 2003, A21.

76. Blood shield laws have also been established to protect blood centers from lawsuits that could put the blood supply in danger. Courts have generally stated that blood shield statutes provide immunity for commercial blood banks and volunteer blood collection agencies. Past lawsuits generally arose from infected blood products transfused into patients prior to the FDA's test for HIV antibodies, which was instituted in 1985. However, sympathy for people who contracted HIV through blood transfusions has not generally resulted in successful litigation. Pieplow, "AIDS, Blood Banks and the Court"; Kelly, "Liability of Blood Banks."

77. Allen, *Talking to Strangers.*

78. Sedgwick, *Epistemology of the Closet,* 40–44.

79. For a brilliant analysis of how discursive and schematic contradictions reinforce power structures, see Ewick and Silbey, *Common Place of Law.*

80. Berlant, *Queen of America,* 16.

81. Ibid., 17.

82. Ibid., 153.

83. This issue will be explored in chapter 4, which examines contemporary medical debates surrounding the blood ban.

84. Various units of the American Association of Blood Banks and America's Blood Centers typically collect the other half.

85. Maistrellis, "American Red Cross," 772.

86. Ibid.

87. Kelly, "Liability of Blood Banks," 466.

88. Maistrellis, "American Red Cross," 778.

89. Ibid., 784.

90. Warner, *Publics and Counterpublics*, 213.

91. Brandzel, "Queering Citizenship," 197.

92. Berlant and Warner, "What Does Queer Theory Teach Us about X?" 345.

CHAPTER 2

1. Although most of this project focuses on the United States' blood policies, the use of the Canadian example is useful for the purposes of this chapter. Because the analysis focuses on the relationship of identity, nation, and citizenship and because the blood bans in Canada and the United States are goaded by similar recommendations and justifications there is little conflict in employing this case. Blood collection agencies in Canada and the United States ask queer men the exact question, with the same deferral policy.

2. Glen McGregor, "Rogers Must ID E-Mail Client: Health Trumps Privacy after Man Claims to Be Actively Gay Blood Donor," *Ottawa Citizen*, June 26, 2002.

3. Ibid.

4. Importantly, if these men were offered tests, this information was not in any of the news stories reported to the public.

5. McGregor, "Rogers Must ID E-Mail Client," A1.

6. Glen McGregor, "Blood Services Stymied by Gay Donor's Taunts," *Ottawa Citizen*, July 28, 2002.

7. Foucault, *History of Sexuality*, 147.

8. Ibid. Ann Laura Stoler has added that Foucault did not look at blood as a definer of "the imperial body and its interior borders." Rather, he examined how "the meanings of blood worked through the technologies of sex and power." *Race and the Education of Desire*, 52.

9. Berlant, "Subject of True Feeling," 47.

10. Mouffe, *Return of the Political*, 60.

11. Of course, countless quotidian acts constitute our citizenship. We drive on the right side of the road, we learn about our communities in the news, and we discuss which leaders would best enhance our world. See Ewick and Silbey, *Common Place of Law*.

12. Allen, *Talking to Strangers*, 136.

13. Foucault, *Power/Knowledge*, 55.

14. Foucault, *History of Sexuality,* 139–145.

15. Foucault, *Discipline and Punish,* 156.

16. McDorman, "Controlling Death," 260.

17. Foucault, *History of Sexuality,* 159.

18. Warner, *Publics and Counterpublics,* 194.

19. Butler, *Gender Trouble,* 23.

20. Butler, "Imitation and Gender Insubordination," 27.

21. Several scholars have challenged Butler's approach, asserting a cloudy relationship between agency and performance. See Jeffreys, "Queer Disappearance." Also, Weston, "Do Clothes Make the Woman?"

22. Keeping one of the basic themes of queer theory in mind, it is important to remember that Butler is not arguing that we necessarily refute everything we understand as natural. Rather, she is attempting to question those discursive forms that normalize one identity at the expense of stigmatizing another.

23. For a thorough analysis of the symbolic import of such systems, see Lévi-Strauss, *Elementary Structures of Kinship.*

24. It should be noted that the Bible always deals explicitly with same-sex "acts," not LGBT relationships in the manner we think of them. Of course, even various sexual acts will carry significantly different meanings today.

25. Schneider, *American Kinship,* 25.

26. Schneider, "Kinship, Nationality, and Religion," 68.

27. Butler, "Is Kinship Always Already Heterosexual?"

28. Schneider, *American Kinship,* 111.

29. Alexander, "Erotic Autonomy," 84.

30. Mosse, *Nationalism and Sexuality,* 29.

31. Butler, "Is Kinship Always Already Heterosexual?"

32. Irons and Guitton, *May It Please the Court,* 370.

33. Nelkin, "Cultural Perspectives on Blood."

34. Proctor, *Racial Hygiene,* 132.

35. Noakes and Pridham, *Documents of Nazism,* 464.

36. Ibid.

37. Of course, blood types do not determine race.

38. Rigg, *Hitler's Jewish Soldiers,* 289.

39. Ibid., 96.

40. The use of the pronoun "he" is employed here intentionally. While there are affiliations between danger and female bisexuality (as it is portrayed in films such as *Basic Instinct*), it is almost always the male bisexual figure who is represented as a threat to the family and the nation in AIDS discourses.

41. Blumfeld, "History/Hysteria," 154–155.

42. Stoler, *Race and the Education of Desire,* 52.

43. Starr, *Blood,* 170.

44. Lemire, *"Miscegenation,"* 144.

45. Love, *One Blood,* 195.

46. In Warner, *Public and Counterpublics,* 188.

47. Marvin and Ingle, *Blood Sacrifice and the Nation,* 23.

48. Bellah, *Habits of the Heart,* 201.

49. See Titmuss, *The Gift Relationship.*

50. Murray, "Poisoned Gift," 222.

51. Ibid.

52. Ibid., 225.

53. Bayer, "Blood and AIDS," 23.

54. Murray, "Poisoned Gift," 232.

55. This is a theme I will return to in chapter 5.

56. On February 19, 2007, George Washington's 275th birthday, President George W. Bush asserted, "On the field of battle, Washington's forces were facing a mighty empire, and the odds against them were overwhelming. The ragged Continental Army lost more battles than it won, suffered waves of desertions, and stood on the brink of disaster many times. Yet George Washington's calm hand and determination kept the cause of independence and the principles of our Declaration alive." Posted on the White House's web site February 19, 2007, at: http://www.whitehouse.gov/news/releases/2007/02/20070219.html. Viewed March 12, 2007.

57. For a full text of Dr. King's "Eulogy for the Young Victims of the Sixteenth Street Baptist Church Bombing," see Carson and Carson, *A Call to Conscience,* 89–100.

58. Marvin and Ingle, *Blood Sacrifice and the Nation,* 11.

59. Ibid., 63.

60. Hewitt, *Mutilating the Body,* 17.

61. I use the words "overt" and "public" here because much sacrifice has been demanded in conflicts such as Iraq. For example, many civil liberties have been sacrificed in the name of advancing the war in Iraq.

62. Rick Tejada-Flores and Judith Ehrlich, "The Good War and Those Who Refused to Fight It" (2000). See the PBS web site at http://www.pbs.org/itvs/thegoodwar/index.html.

63. Love, *One Blood,* 187.

64. Douglas, *Purity and Danger,* 52.

65. Horner and Anderson, "Integration of Homosexuals into the Armed Forces," 253–254.

66. Koegel, "Lessons Learned," 144.

67. National Defense Research Institute, *Sexual Orientation,* 454.

68. Kauth and Landis, "Applying Lessons Learned," 94.

69. National Defense Research Institute, *Sexual Orientation,* 372.

70. "Do Draft, Do Tell," *Advocate,* February 18, 2003.

71. Marvin and Ingle, *Blood Sacrifice and the Nation,* 108.

72. National Defense Research Institute, *Sexual Orientation,* 370.

73. Yingling, *AIDS and the National Body,* 32.

74. Butler, *Excitable Speech,* 14.

75. Yingling, *AIDS and the National Body,* 16.

76. Patton, "From Nation to Family," 279.

77. Ibid., 287.

78. Morrow, "AIDS and Immigration," 278.

79. On World AIDS Day, December 1, 2006, President Bush issued an executive order granting a "categorical Waiver" to "HIV-positive people entering the U.S. for tourism or business reasons for up to 60 days." At the time of this writing, however, that stringent regulation remains in place. A Senate bill that was expected to be signed by President Bush the week of July 28, 2008, would change the restriction. As of late fall 2008, the travel ban is still in place. See Paul Kidd, "U.S. Plans to Ease HIV Travel Restrictions," *Positive Living,* December 21, 2006.

80. Brier, "Immigrant Infection," 254.

81. Ibid., 256.

82. Again, this is not to suggest that all heterosexuals can donate blood. Many heterosexuals who have lived outside of the country, for example, cannot. However, these conditions are usually temporary and are not related to the stigmatization of their identity.

83. In contrast, critics such as Warner have warned that investing so much time and energy in issues such as gays in the military diverts attention from the problems of AIDS. He explains that "with its vision of patriotic death, its vision of national loyalties trumping all other partisan ties, the military issue almost seems designed to produce amnesia about AIDS." But critics and activists need not engage in the kind of amnesia described by Warner to delimit the rhetorical structures that intimately link notions of AIDS with nationalistic discourses when it comes to issues such as "gays in the military" or the blood ban. *Publics and Counterpublics,* 239.

84. Butler, *Excitable Speech,* 114.

85. Yingling, *AIDS and the National Body,* 39.

86. Joseph, *Nomadic Identities,* 4.

87. See Harvard Law Review, *Sexual Orientation and the Law.* Also Kaplan, *Sexual Justice.*

88. Florida Legislative Investigation Committee, "Homosexuality and Citizenship in Florida," 1.

89. Ibid.

90. Ibid.

91. Hall, "On Postmodernism and Articulation," 141.

92. Grossberg, *We Gotta Get Out of This Place,* 54.

93. Slack, "Theory and Method of Articulation," 125.

94. Of course, the development of queer theory itself was a result of the gay and lesbian rights movement. Groups of scholars sought to resist the degree to which gays, lesbians, and other sexual minorities were "normalizing" the manner in which we constructed sexual identities.

95. Mann, "Has Globalization Ended the Rise of the Nation-State?" 144–145.

96. Goffman, *Stigma,* 121.

97. Ibid., 122.

98. Yingling, *AIDS and the National Body,* 45.

99. Kristeva, *Powers of Horror,* 4.

100. Ibid., 15.

101. Young, "Abjection and Oppression," 209.

102. Marvin and Ingle, *Blood Sacrifice and the Nation,* 8.

103. Warner, *Publics and Counterpublics,* 220.

104. Of course, if these were female detractors, "Jane Doe" would have been the name of choice.

105. Dyer, *Seven,* 45.

106. Kevin Spacey played the role of "Jonathan Doe" in the film *Seven.* His character murdered victims in manners that were connected to the seven deadly sins such as gluttony, wrath, and, of course, pride.

107. Kristeva, *Strangers to Ourselves,* 13.

108. The next chapter will highlight specifically how these contradictions are deployed to help reinvigorate the power of the state.

109. See Sedgwick, *Epistemology of the Closet.*

110. Again, this is not to imply that all things are outside the realm of human understanding. Rather, it is to illustrate the discursive attempts made to sharpen the contrast between the "known" and the "unknown."

111. Alwood, *Straight News,* 10.

CHAPTER 3

1. The National Gay Task Force did not become the National Gay and Lesbian Task Force until 1985.

2. Shilts, *Band,* 221.

3. The name AIDS was originally agreed upon at a meeting called by the Center for Disease Control in July 1982.

4. Of course, being a television production, it ignores any number of significant facts. This includes the point that it had been a scant seven years since the American Psychological Association had taken homosexuality off its list of psychological disorders and further stigmatizing gay people was an important concern.

5. Triechler, *How to Have Theory in an Epidemic.*

6. Marita Sturken, *Tangled Memories,* 179.

7. For more on the contradictory forms that mark discourses of homosexuality, see Sedgwick, *Epistomolgy of the Closet.*

8. This is not to say that such archives do not exist, but that these agencies, at this time, either did not have them or elected not to release them.

9. Shilts himself acknowledged using only the *Philadelphia Inquirer,* the *New York Native,* interviews, and press releases to reconstruct the happenings of the meeting. *Band,* 613.

10. Zelizer, "Reading the Past," 214.

11. Foucault, *Birth of the Clinic,* 25.

12. Shilts, *Band,* 220.

13. Although *Band* and *Red Gold* are the most explicit texts that feature the blood ban, queer donors were hinted at in other cultural texts throughout the 1980s and early 1990s. The LGBT television scholar Stephen Tropiano, for instance, notes that "many sitcoms focused on an adult heterosexual or a child who became infected through a blood transfusion." For example, *The Golden Girls* featured an episode when the naïvely pure of heart character Rose Nylund (played by Betty White) had a scare after a blood transfusion. While it is never overtly stated that the donor was gay the text allowed the unknown donor to be read as such. White's character suggests that she is undeserving of the scare because she is "safe" and that her sexually promiscuous roommate Blanche (played by Rue McClanahan) should have to suffer the anxiety instead. The connection between promiscuity and AIDS is made and challenged, diverted to bodies not typically associated with HIV infection (elderly white women). *Prime Time Closet,* 235.

14. Sturken, *Tangled Memories,* 177.

15. Crimp, *Melancholia and Moralism,* 125.

16. Ibid., 46.

17. Ibid., 119.

18. Ibid., 60.

19. Watney, *Policing Desire.*

20. There are films that are not as dependent on marketing values. Several forms of independent and documentary film, for example, are often free from such constraints, though these divisions are increasingly rare.

21. Hariman, "Prudence in the Twenty-first Century," 288.

22. In his detailing of the original blood deferral policies, for example, Ronald Bayer asserted that the Public Health Service set forth their "'prudent' proposals" despite the objections by gay lobbyists. "Blood and AIDS," 25.

23. Nelson, "Prudence as Republican Politics," 230.

24. Lipsitz, *Time Passages,* 5.

25. It should be noted that media forms, such as the docudramas explored in this chapter, do not have to purposely seek to reinforce the ideology of the dominate powers. Indeed, the narrative structure of popular culture forges a specific kind of audience appeal, one that seeks to reinforce what viewers believe, even if these values are packaged in purportedly novel information.

26. Bodnar, *Remaking America,* 15.

27. Taylor, *Archive and the Repertoire,* 16–33.

28. Oravec, "Fanny Wright," 190.

29. Ibid., 205.

30. Sturken, *Tangled Memories,* 176.

31. But for doubters, please see Triechler, *How to Have Theory in an Epidemic;* Crimp, *AIDS: Cultural Analysis.*

32. Susan Ager, "AIDS: Many Questions, Few Answers," *Detroit Free Press,* October 6, 1985, B1.

33. Nelson, "Prudence as Republican Politics," 244.

34. Starr, *Blood,* 278.

35. It should be noted that this motif of the red and white lights is a constant on this particular portion of the series. The video opens with this artistry and employs it several other times through the duration of the program.

36. Starr, *Blood,* 277.

37. Ibid., 321.

38. From *Red Gold.* This particular quote was taken from the third part of the series titled *Tainted Blood.*

39. Starr, *Blood,* 323–324.

40. Ibid., 278.

41. Ibid., 277.

42. Ibid., 273; Shilts, *Band,* 220. This scene is also featured in the movie version of *Band.*

43. Larry Martz, "A New Panic over AIDS," *Newsweek,* March 30, 1987, 18.

44. Starr, *Blood,* 277.

45. Ibid., 336.

46. Corea, *Invisible Epidemic,* 265.

47. Editorial, "Denying the AIDS Danger: Three Decades Later, Many Educated Gays Ignore the Risks. Why?" *Ottawa Citizen,* July 30, 2002, A12.

48. America's Blood Centers, "ABC Communications Department E-Newsletter," January 16, 2004, 2.

49. Sabin Russell, "Warnings from the Scientific Community," *San Francisco Chronicle,* July 14, 2002, A3.

50. African Americans and Latinos are often not a part of the educational campaigns mentioned in the editorial, which tend to be directed toward white gay men or heterosexual communities. Associated Press, "Few Men Aware They're Infected," *Gazette,* July 9, 2002, A1.

51. Summerrise and DeCarlo, *What Are Heterosexual Men's HIV Prevention Needs?;* Harris Interactive, "Six of Ten Heterosexual Adults in America Have Not Been Tested for HIV, New National Survey Finds" (2003); available from http://www.harrisinteractive.com/news/allnewsbydate.asp?NewsID=714.

52. To avoid totalizing, a number of gay men did oppose efforts such as closing the bathhouses. However, this image ignores the many voices that proposed other paths of action.

53. Starr, *Blood,* 296.

54. Ibid., 269.

55. There is wide consensus that the government failed to more actively speak with a singular voice that could have prevented an undetermined amount of infections. Likewise, the blood industry could have been more active in their donor screening procedures. Dr. Oscar Ratnoff suggested that hemophiliacs suspend use of Factor VIII and use "safer cryoprecipitate, made from pools of ten donors or less." Industry officials and hemophiliac doctors opposed such measures, arguing that hemophiliacs

would face similar rates of HIV infection. Such predictions turned out to be false. See ibid., 272.

56. In June 1983 at the World Hemophilia Federation's annual meeting officials passed a resolution stating hemophiliacs should continue using Factor VIII, despite the fact they knew several businesses had not yet begun taking measures to detect HIV in the blood supply. Some countries such as Britain, France, and Japan actually increased their use of the substance. American organizations such as the National Hemophilia Foundation had also promoted the continued use of blood products, but their ties to industries that benefited from the sale of such products seriously damaged their reputation, sparking widespread protests at conventions.

57. Nelkin, "Cultural Perspectives," 287.

58. Kirp, "The Politics of Blood," 297.

59. Ibid., 308.

60. Women can be carriers of the genes that cause hemophilia, but are almost never diagnosed with the actual disorder. About one out of every five thousand men is born hemophiliac.

61. Kirp, "The Politics of Blood," 297–299.

62. Ibid., 310.

63. Starr, *Blood,* 272.

64. Ibid., 278.

65. Starr cites the case of Dana Kuhn, a married man with mild hemophilia who had been given an injection of Factor VIII after injuring himself during a basketball game. Because it was the only time that Kuhn had ever been given Factor VIII, doctors were hesitant to give him an AIDS test. It was Kuhn who insisted he be tested for AIDS, ultimately discovering that he was positive. Tragically, Kuhn passed AIDS on to his wife and she died just one year later.

66. Fausto-Sterling, "How to Build a Man," 132.

67. I do not dispute the fact that Factor VIII has helped thousands of hemophiliacs attain a more humane and healthy life. I am simply articulating the point that the word "normal" is central to the discourse employed by hemophiliac activists and health officials alike.

68. Bayer, "Blood and AIDS," 41.

69. Ibid., 45.

70. Cited in ibid.

71. This has been noticed in the medical community as well. See ibid.

72. Institute of Medicine, *HIV and the Blood Supply,* 104.

73. Ibid., 122.

74. Ibid., 124.

75. Ibid., 111, 22.

76. Scott Lively and Kevin Abrams, *The Pink Swastika: Homosexuality in the Nazi Party* (Keiser, OR: Founders Publishing, 1997), 210.

77. Nelson, "Prudence as Republican Politics," 251–253.

78. Mosse, *Nationalism and Sexuality,* 25.

79. Phelan, *Unmarked,* 135.

80. Editorial, "Denying the AIDS Danger," A12.

81. Glied, "Circulation of Blood," 331.

82. Ibid., 330.

83. See Ports, "Needed."

84. Institute of Medicine, *HIV and the Blood Supply,* 105.

85. Ibid., 122.

CHAPTER 4

1. This was true when I first looked at the page in March 2001 and when I checked the site over seven years later on July 19, 2008. The site can be found at http://chapters.redcross.org/ca/norcal/donor/faq.html.

2. Although the FDA mandates the ban, a large amount of the information used in the decision-making process comes from the CDC.

3. Condit, "Birth of Understanding," 324.

4. *St. Petersburg Times,* "Erring on the Side of Safe Blood," September 16, 2000. Emphasis mine.

5. Prelli, "Rhetorical Logic," 317.

6. Lyne and Howe, "Punctuated Equilibria," 132; Smith, *Scandalous Knowledge.*

7. Duster, *Backdoor to Eugenics,* 37.

8. Young, *Inclusion and Democracy,* 86.

9. Duster, *Backdoor to Eugenics;* Proctor, *Racial Hygiene;* Drescher, "I'm Your Handyman."

10. Jones, *Bad Blood,* 21.

11. Brookey, *Reinventing the Male Homosexual.*

12. For example, see Hamer and Copeland, *Science of Desire.*

13. See, for example, Burkett, *Gravest Show on Earth;* Crimp, *AIDS: Cultural Analysis;* Crimp, *Melancholia and Moralism;* Dowsett, *Practicing Desire;* Epstein, *Impure Science;* Patton, *Sex and Germs;* Patton, *Inventing AIDS;* Patton, *Fatal Advice.*

14. See Reeves, "Rhetoric and the AIDS Virus Hunt."

15. Crimp, *AIDS Demographics.*

16. Burkett, *Gravest Show on Earth,* 275.

17. Erica Goode, "Certain Words Can Trip Up AIDS Grants, Scientists Say," *New York Times,* April 18, 2003, A10.

18. Nicholas Kristof, "No Time to Get Squeamish," *New York Times,* May 9, 2003, A31.

19. Burkett, *Gravest Show on Earth,* 175.

20. BPAC, *67th Meeting,* 246.

21. Why the FDA waited over fourteen months following this meeting to announce this decision was not clear. A representative I spoke with the day after the announcement said there was no rationale for why the decision was made public when it was.

22. Two distinguishing factors matter most when factoring the differences between the two policy-making meetings, both of which will be highlighted in this chapter. First is the introduction of Nucleic Acid Testing in 1999, which has substantially closed the so-called window period following HIV infection that prevents the virus from being detected. Studies involving NAT were not seriously considered in 2000. The second factor is the cultural changes that had transpired around LGBT rights in America between the years 2000 and 2006.

23. For treatments of deliberations, their limitations, and their potential, see Ivie, *Democracy and America's War on Terror;* Young, *Intersecting Voices;* Young, *Inclusion and Democracy;* Benhabib, *Democracy and Difference;* Guttman, *Democracy and Disagreement.*

24. Young, *Intersecting Voices,* 62.

25. Burke, *Language as Symbolic Action,* 44–62.

26. Plummer, *Intimate Citizenship,* 28–29.

27. Ivie, *Democracy and America's War on Terror,* 196–197.

28. BPAC, *57th Meeting,* 55.

29. Ibid., 200.

30. Ibid., 53.

31. A "seroconversion" means the virus is no longer dormant and can be detected through standard scientific measures because HIV antibodies are present. In technical terms, it means that one has developed "specific antibodies to an infectious microorganism in response to either natural infection or vaccination." Ibid., 61.

32. Ibid., 74–75.

33. Dayton preempted the obvious problems of tracing queer donors. He pondered for the committee, "Where do we get this number from? Simply put, we took calculations of known male homosexual behavior and what percentage of the population exhibited or pursued 'MSM' behavior, and there is data on what percentage of those have abstained for various time periods." Ibid., 58.

34. Ibid., 63.

35. Ibid., 74.

36. FDA, *Workshop,* 87.

37. Ibid., 201.

38. Ibid., 202.

39. Ibid., 203.

40. Ibid., 254, 333.

41. Of one study, Doll explained that "26 percent of the men responded that because of these new treatments, they were less concerned about becoming HIV infected and this was about a year ago, say, maybe 14 months ago, I believe, 13 to 15 percent of the men stated they would be willing to take a chance at becoming infected or had already done so because of the availability of new treatments."

42. BPAC, *57th Meeting,* 82.

43. Ibid., 72.

44. Ibid., 82.

45. BPAC, *67th Meeting*, 260.

46. Ibid., 237.

47. For one such study, see Harris Interactive, *Six of Ten Heterosexual Adults in America Have Not Been Tested for HIV, New National Survey Finds* (2003); available from http://www.harrisinteractive.com/news/allnewsbydate.asp?NewsID=714.

48. FDA, *Workshop*, 60.

49. Ibid., 61.

50. Despite this articulation, there were times when the doctors were more considerate of some variables than they were at the previous two meetings. Van der Poel, for example, took the monogamy of queer men into account when focusing on Hepatitis B. The doctor reported: "In MSMs there were 6 cases in 2004 in people with a steady partner and 82 in people with a casual partner." Ibid., 82.

51. Ibid., 266–267.

52. BPAC, *67th Meeting*, 192.

53. Yingling, *AIDS and the National Body*, 25.

54. Martin, *Flexible Bodies*, 133.

55. Ibid., 97.

56. BPAC, *67th Meeting*, 162.

57. BPAC, *57th Meeting*, 170.

58. Ibid., 155.

59. FDA, *Workshop*, 122, 39.

60. BPAC, *67th Meeting*, 165.

61. BPAC, *57th Meeting*, 166.

62. BPAC, *67th Meeting*, 181, 86, 96, 289, 90.

63. Ibid., 182. Emphasis in the text is mine.

64. Ibid., 187, 84.

65. FDA, *Workshop*, 376.

66. Ibid., 378.

67. Ibid., 386.

68. Ibid., 387.

69. Smith, *Scandalous Knowledge*, 58.

70. BPAC, *57th Meeting*, 91–92.

71. The issue of STD clinical data again surfaced at the 2006 meeting, though it was not transparent how much of the information being presented came from such locations. McKenna expressed concern with the data collected from STD clinics, saying, "These are high risk populations, of course. These are people who are being tested for HIV and attending clinics that have counseling and testing services." He pointed out that one of his studies was not a household survey. "These are persons attending venues where we know individuals are going to be at very high risk." FDA, *Workshop*, 105, 107.

72. Doll could be suggesting these are places in the "real world" not hampered with the same baggage that accompanies STD clinics. BPAC, *57th Meeting*, 92.

73. Age surfaced a couple of times during the 2006 meeting, most noticeably when McKenna was addressing the issue of HIV rates in the queer community. "The older they were, there was decreasing unawareness of their infection." FDA, *Workshop,* 106.

74. BPAC, *57th Meeting,* 99.

75. Ibid.

76. Not only do "MSMs" supposedly harbor dangerous infections that are within the realm of standard scientific medical practices, they are also discussed in relation to diseases that could pass through the blood supply undetected by scientific measures. Dr. Nelson reports, "There has been a recent report in Clinical Infectious Disease of an AIDS patient that never seroconverted, and that is almost unique, but cases have been reported."

77. FDA, *Workshop,* 144.

78. Ibid., 330.

79. Patton, *Sex and Germs,* 131.

80. BPAC, *67th Meeting,* 227.

81. Jane Brody, "Abstinence-Only: Does It Work?" *New York Times,* June 1, 2004; Maggie Fox, "Abstinence Education Doesn't Work," *Reuters,* April 14, 2007.

82. For excellent critiques of such risks, see Warner, *The Trouble with Normal,* 195–218, and Halperin, *What Do Gay Men Want?*

83. BPAC, *67th Meeting,* 304.

84. Ibid., 314.

85. Again, this is not to suggest that MSM could never be a productive term. In this context, however, it offers an avenue around identity that works to the disadvantage of queer men.

86. In Cohen, *Boundaries,* 107.

87. For more on the power of remaining unmarked, see Phelan, *Unmarked.*

88. Dowsett, *Practicing Desire,* 34.

89. Moore, *Beyond Shame,* 158.

90. Boykin, *Beyond the Down Low,* 91–92.

91. Daryn Kagan and Linda Yee, "U.S. FDA Considers Lifting Ban on Homosexual Men Donating Blood," *CNN Morning News,* September 13, 2000.

92. BPAC, *67th Meeting,* 220.

93. Ibid., 200, 38.

94. Ibid., 225.

95. Ibid., 299.

96. Ibid., 300. Emphasis mine.

97. BPAC, *57th Meeting,* 219.

98. Ibid., 221.

99. Ibid., 114.

100. Ibid., 210.

101. Ibid., 263.

102. Ibid., 264–265.

103. Ibid., 225.

104. BPAC, *67th Meeting*, 193.

105. Like many votes in the year 2000, it was a close call. The committee voted 7–6 in favor of upholding the ban.

106. Gene Randall and Rusty Dornin, "Gay Community Says It's Time to Lift Ban on Homosexual Blood Donations," *CNN Worldview*, January 13, 2000.

107. BPAC, *67th Meeting*, 228.

108. Special thanks to the American Association of Blood Banks for confirming this information.

109. Patton, *Sex and Germs*, 39.

110. Starr, *Blood*, 349–350.

111. Rousseau, "Discourse on Political Economy," 61.

112. FDA, *Workshop*, 91, 180.

113. BPAC, *67th Meeting*, 235.

114. In 2006 the American Red Cross publicly supported the relaxing of blood-donor deferral measures lodged against queer men to one year for those men that are sexually active.

115. BPAC, *67th Meeting*, 257.

116. Ibid., 260.

117. Ibid., 263.

118. Gramsci, *Prison Notebooks*, 242.

119. Bob Roehr, *The Gift of Life: Gay Men and US Blood Donation Policy*, Liberty Education Forum, October 30, 2002.

120. Mary McLachlin, "Three Groups Denounce Blood Drive Contracts," *Palm Beach Post*, January 24, 2003.

121. Starr, *Blood*, 355–356.

122. Foucault, *Discipline and Punish*, 221.

123. FDA, *Workshop*, 329.

124. Ibid., 338.

125. Ibid., 340.

126. Matt King, "FDA Will Not Lift Ban So Gays Can Give Blood," *San Jose Mercury News*, March 14, 2007.

127. Special thanks to several people who helped in the development of this chapter. Representatives from the American Association of Blood Banks and the Indiana Blood Center provided important information regarding blood regulation and legal details. Indiana University law professor Susan Williams had interesting comments to share and made important legal clarifications during the initial draft of this chapter.

CHAPTER 5

1. Warner, *Publics and Counterpublics*, 76.

2. Allen, *Talking to Strangers*, 10.

3. Ibid., 41.

4. On the rhetorical force of "equality," see Condit and Lucaites, *Crafting Equality*.

5. For discussions of identity politics, see Michaels, *The Trouble with Diversity,* 1–20; Anderson, *Way We Argue Now,* 21–66; Gitlin, *Twilight of Common Dreams;* Slagle, "In Defense of Queer Nation," 85–102.

6. There are likely a number of men who admit to being gay and leave the blood center quietly because of shame, embarrassment, and anger.

7. Scott, *Domination and the Arts of Resistance,* 199.

8. Kelley, "Not What We Seem," 111.

9. In concentrating on queer men, I do not intend to undermine the support and subversive actions of those who do not identify as such. Many heterosexuals, lesbians, and bisexual women do not support these policies.

10. Morris, "Responsibility of the Critic," 263.

11. As mentioned in the previous chapter, Dr. Michael Busch told a 2006 workshop sponsored by the FDA that blood centers only deal with one or two HIV-positive donations a year and those usually come from heterosexuals. Since the implementation of the Nucleic Acid Testing in San Francisco "there have been four really proven HIV transfusion transmissions missed by mini-pool NAT." Busch said, "I just wanted to point out that none of these were MSM, or acknowledged MSM. Two of them were women with heterosexual infection and one was a male who, on follow-up extensive interview, denied MSM activity. So, what is getting through now is not related to MSM." FDA, *Workshop,* 202–203.

12. Warner, *Publics and Counterpublics,* 122.

13. Spradlin, "Price of 'Passing,'" 598.

14. Blackmer, "Veils of the Law," 63.

15. Ginsberg, "Politics of Passing," 2.

16. Robinson, "It Takes One to Know One," 721. See also Morris, "Pink Herring," 228–244.

17. Ginsberg, "Politics of Passing," 2.

18. Among other places, passing remains a necessity in many sport cultures. It is also a necessity in many immigrant cultures and religions. Lest passing be dismissed as no longer vital to queer life, one need only revisit the 2004 elections when eleven states passed amendments banning gay marriage. In those states where the votes against gays and lesbians were especially high, queers continue to live in a volatile world where being out and proud is not always an option.

19. Lahiri, "Performing Identity," 411.

20. Squires and Brouwer, "In/Discernible Bodies," 287.

21. Shugart, "Performing Ambiguity," 30–54; Sloop, "Disciplining the Transgendered," 165–189; Squires and Brouwer, "In/Discernible Bodies," 283–310.

22. Warner, *Publics and Counterpublics,* 122.

23. To avoid totalizing, I do not mean to imply that all men have similar motives when passing or protesting.

24. See, for example, Douglas, *Purity and Danger.*

25. FDA, *Workshop,* 329.

26. Andrew Keegan, "FDA Meeting Revisits Ban on Gay Blood Donors," *Southern*

Voice, March 10, 2006, http://www.sovo.com/print.cfm?content_id=5077 (accessed June 14, 2007).

27. De Certeau, *Practice of Everyday Life,* 5.

28. Warner, *Publics and Counterpublics,* 121.

29. The interviews were undertaken according to a plan approved specifically by the IRB at Indiana University (#03–7891). Volunteers were found by posting announcements on several e-mail listservs. All of the interviews were completed by me in person or by telephone and each took approximately forty-five minutes to complete. The names of the respondents have been disguised by the use of first names only and these are not their actual names. While there was a core set of questions, the interviews were open-ended so that the respondents could best characterize their experiences with the donation policies and feelings toward agencies that mandate the ban. Unlike many university studies, the majority of these men were not students. As such, their ages, geographic locations, and attitudes toward blood, sexuality, and HIV varied. As the men offered their information, it became apparent that altruism, not civil disobedience, largely guided their practices. This led me back to materials about passing and protesting. Especially in relation to passing, the men's responses altered the ways in which these tropes were traditionally understood in the literature.

30. For more on the felt duty associated with "coming out," see Patton, "Tremble," 173.

31. Allen, *Talking to Strangers,* 29.

32. This was mentioned during the 2006 conference on donor deferral policies sponsored by the FDA. FDA, *Workshop.*

33. Warner, *Publics and Counterpublics,* 75.

34. Bell, *Ritual Theory.*

35. Institute of Medicine, *HIV and the Blood Supply: An Analysis of Crisis Decision Making,* ed. Lauren Leveton, Harold C. Sox, and Michael Stoto (Washington, D.C.: National Academy Press, 1995), 111, 122.

36. The blood ban is likely given little attention in both the popular and queer presses because it is offered scant attention by major LGBT organizations. Being closely associated with AIDS and not an explicit "civil right," the issue of blood donation is often seen as too culturally taboo.

37. Scott, *Domination and the Arts of Resistance,* 188.

38. For a critique of reproductive futurism, please see Lee Edelman's *No Future.*

39. This will come as little surprise to those familiar with Foucault's work on discipline. However, one should not assume that simply because some men withheld from donation that their previous donations were less useful in challenging cultural assumptions about the safety of their blood. Nor does it suggest all of the men in this study stopped donating. On discipline, see Foucault, *Discipline and Punish;* Sloop, *Disciplining Gender;* Ehlers, "Hidden in Plain Sight," 313–334.

40. There are several Red Cross regions that share information with one another. According to a Red Cross employee I spoke with, the organization is currently working on a system that will allow blood centers across the country to exchange infor-

mation. While individual centers record only the length of time a person is deferred, the regional centers have access to the specific reason why people cannot contribute blood.

41. For an excellent account of queer life in rural areas, as well as compelling examples of transgender passing, see Halberstam, *In a Queer Time and Place.*

42. For extended analyses of the gays in the military debate, see Herek, Jobe, and Carey, *Out in Force;* Scott and Stanley, *Gays and Lesbians in the Military.*

43. Please see chapter 4 for an extended discussion of the evidence employed by the government and benevolent organizations such as the Red Cross.

44. Butler, *Undoing Gender,* 57–74.

45. Just as it is always problematic to infer that gay men are HIV positive, it is also dangerous to stereotype blood workers as demonic minions. Indeed, perhaps one of the more troubling elements of these interviews was the extent to which blood-center volunteers had so little information about the policies they were enforcing. While queer men can protest at the site of the civic ritual, those they are challenging have no say in the policy itself.

46. Sedgwick, "Queer Performativity."

47. Lahiri, "Performing Identity," 412.

48. Many of the "older" men interviewed had witnessed substantial changes over the past several decades. They insisted that changes to the policy would occur eventually, being a matter of time before scientific evidence, popular opinion, or monetary reasons forced a revision of the questionnaire. Some, such as Jacob, believed the policies would change because of severe shortages or because of money. "I think it will come down to the dollar, not right or wrong. I kind of put the Red Cross in the same place that I put the Boy Scouts. For me, they're going to need to make some choices and there will be some consequences to those choices . . . but it's their choice to make."

49. Kristeva, *Strangers to Ourselves,* 7.

50. There is a difference between the blood and bone marrow policies. A man who has had sex with another man one time in the past five years is deferred from acting as a marrow donor. Clearly, this still eliminates scores of healthy donors. As with the blood-donor questionnaire, sex is never defined.

51. Of course, this does not include women who are omitted for reasons noted on the questionnaire.

52. On the relationship among hierarchy, identification, and scapegoating, see Burke, *Philosophy of Literary Form,* 191–220.

53. Although some men reported negative experiences with blood-center employees, most agreed that, even when turned away, the workers were still friendly and professional, albeit uncomfortable. As Simon, the man who attempts to donate at least once a year, observed, "Well, most of the time, I mean the poor people they're just there to draw your blood." Thomas, who had organized the blood drive for hundreds of people at his place of employment, said the blood-center worker joked with him about not being able to give. "They did compliment me on the amount of blood I had inspired people to give." Matthew says he was in a situation where the blood collection worker

happened to be gay. He explained, "The people who I dealt with during that experience were very kind. I was pissed at the rules, I wasn't mad at the people. In fact, the guy and the woman taking blood, they were both very nice and they were like 'if it were up to us we would allow you to do it.'"

54. Scott, *Seeing Like a State.*

55. Joey Diguglielmo, "Blood Boiling Over Ban," *Washington Blade,* April 7, 2007, http://www.washingtonblade.com/2007/4–27/view/actionalert/10498.cfm (accessed July 8, 2007); "New Hampshire Students Protest Gay Blood Ban," *365gay.com,* April 22, 2005, http://www.365gay.com/newscon05/04/042205blood.htm (accessed June 14, 2007); Steven Bodzin, "Students Tap New Vein of Gay Issue," *Los Angeles Times,* July 10, 2005, http://www.aegis.com/news/lt/2005/LT050704.html (accessed June 14, 2007); Marie-Jo Mont-Reynaud, "Banned from the Blood Bank," *Stanford Daily,* May 25, 2006, http://daily.stanford.edu/article/2006/5/25/bannedFromTheBloodBank (accessed June 14, 2007).

56. "Students Protest Ban on Gay Blood," *Advocate.com,* October 19, 2006, http://www.advocate.com/print_article_ektid37683.asp (accessed June 14, 2007).

CHAPTER 6

1. Advocate, *College Blood Drive Canceled over Exclusion of Gays,* May 20, 2003.

2. Ibid.

3. On the limits of "tolerance," see Brown, *Regulating Aversion.*

4. The original e-mail spelled "judgment" as "judgement." While this is a less frequently used form of the word, it is an acceptable spelling.

5. See chapter 4 for an extend discussion of the window period.

6. Examples of this scholarship might include Butler, *Bodies That Matter;* Foucault, *History of Sexuality;* Gramsci, *Prison Notebooks;* Scott, *Domination and the Arts of Resistance.*

7. Cruikshank, "Cultural Politics," 76.

8. Plummer, *Telling Sexual Stories,* 148.

9. Weeks, *Invented Moralities,* 153.

10. Ibid.

11. For an extended analysis of these gendered metaphors, see Martin, *Egg and the Sperm.*

12. Jonathan Curiel, "Gay Male Blood Donor Ban Called Unfair; S.F. Supervisor Wants FDA to Change Policy," *San Francisco Chronicle,* January 7, 2000, A20.

13. Arendt, *Origins of Totalitarianism,* 17.

14. Douglas Starr, "Relax the Ban on Gay Blood Donors," *Los Angeles Times,* April 30, 2000, M2.

15. Reuters, "Blood Donor Pool May Be Overestimated," *MSNBC.com,* August 14, 2007, http://www.msnbc.msn.com/id/20268581/from/RS.5 (accessed August 14, 2007).

16. BPAC, *67th Meeting,* 301.

17. See especially Duggan, "Queering the State"; Warner, *Fear of a Queer Planet*.

18. Ibid.

19. Young, *Intersecting Voices,* 73.

20. See http://bloodsense.blogspot.com.

21. Sarah Varney, "Blood Donation Rules Roil California Campuses," *All Things Considered,* June 11, 2008.

22. Joel Aleccia, "As Donations Decline, Nation Needs Young Blood," *MSNBC.com,* May 20, 2008, http://www.msnbc.msn.com/id/24730183 (accessed May 20, 2008).

23. San Jose State University, "Blood Drive Suspension Update," April 14, 2008, http://www.sjsu.edu/news/releases/releases_detail.jsp?id=2815 (accessed June 24, 2008).

24. See, for example, Mouffe, *Democratic Paradox*.

Works Cited

Alexander, M. Jacqui. "Erotic Autonomy as a Politics of Decolonization: An Anatomy of Feminist and State Practice in the Bahamas Tourist Economy." In *Feminist Genealogies, Colonial Legacies, Democratic Futures,* ed. M. Jacqui Alexander and Chandra Talpade Mohanty, 63–100. New York: Routledge, 1997.

Allen, Danielle. *Talking to Strangers: Anxieties of Citizenship since Brown v. Board of Education.* Chicago: University of Chicago Press, 2004.

Althusser, Louis. *Politics and History: Montesquieu, Rousseau, Marx.* Trans. Ben Brewster. 1972. London: Verso, 2007.

Alwood, Edward. *Straight News: Gays, Lesbians, and the News Media.* New York: Columbia University Press, 1996.

American Red Cross. "September 11, 2001: Unprecedented Events, Unprecedented Response. A Review of the American Red Cross' Response in the Past Year," 2001.

And the Band Played On. Dir. Roger Spottiswoode. HBO Home Video, 1993. Videocassette.

Anderson, Amanda. *The Way We Argue Now: A Study in the Cultures of Theory.* Princeton, NJ: Princeton University Press, 2006.

Arendt, Hannah. *The Origins of Totalitarianism.* New York: Harcourt Brace Jovanovich, 1951.

Asen, Robert, and Daniel Brouwer. *Counterpublics and the State.* Albany: State University of New York Press, 2001.

Bayer, Ronald. "Blood and AIDS in America: Science, Politics, and the Making of an Iatrogenic Catastrophe." In *Blood Feuds: AIDS, Blood, and the Politics of Medical Disaster,* ed. Eric Feldman and Ronald Bayer, 19–58. New York: Oxford University Press, 1999.

Bell, Catherine. *Ritual Theory, Ritual Practice.* New York: Oxford University Press, 1992.

Bellah, Robert N., Richard Madsen, William M. Sullivan, Ann Swidler, and Steven M. Tipton. *Habits of the Heart: Individualism and Commitment in American Life.* Berkeley and Los Angeles: University of California Press, 1985.

Benhabib, Seyla, ed. *Democracy and Difference: Contesting the Boundaries of the Political.* Princeton, NJ: Princeton University Press, 1996.

Berlant, Lauren. *The Queen of America Goes to Washington City: Essays on Sex and Citizenship.* Durham, NC: Duke University Press, 1997.

———. "The Subject of True Feeling: Pain, Privacy, and Politics." In *Cultural Studies and Political Theory,* ed. Jodi Dean, 42–62. Ithaca, NY: Cornell University Press, 2000.

Berlant, Lauren, and Michael Warner. "Sex in Public." *Critical Inquiry* 24 (1998): 547–566.

———. "What Does Queer Theory Teach Us about X?" *Publication of the Modern Language Association* 110 (1995): 343–349.

Blackmer, Corinne. "The Veils of the Law: Race and Sexuality in Nella Larsen's *Passing.*" *College Literature* 22 (1995): 50–68.

Blood Products Advisory Committee. *57th Meeting of the Blood Products Advisory Committee.* December 11, 1997.

———. *67th Meeting of the Blood Products Advisory Committee.* September 14, 2000.

Blumfeld, Warren. "History/Hysteria: Parallel Representations of Jews and Gays, Lesbians, and Bisexuals." In *Queer Studies: A Lesbian, Gay, Bisexual, and Transgender Anthology,* ed. Brett Beemyn and Mickey Eliason, 146–162. New York: New York University Press, 1996.

Bodnar, John. *Remaking America: Public Memory, Commemoration, and Patriotism in the Twentieth Century.* Princeton, NJ: Princeton University Press, 1992.

Bordo, Susan. "The Body and the Production of Femininity: A Feminist Appropriation of Foucault." In *Gender/Body/Knowledge: Feminist Reconstructions of Being and Knowing,* ed. Alison Jaggar and Susan Bordo, 13–33. New Brunswick, NJ: Rutgers University Press, 1992.

Boykin, Keith. *Beyond the Down Low: Sex, Lies, and Denial in Black America.* New York: Carroll and Graf Publishers, 2005.

Brandzel, Amy. "Queering Citizenship? Same-Sex Marriage and the State." *GLQ* 11 (2005): 171–204.

Brier, Jennifer. "The Immigrant Infection: Images of Race, Nation, and Contagion in the Public Debates on AIDS and Immigration." In *Modern American Queer History,* ed. Allida M. Black, 253–270. Philadelphia: Temple University Press, 2001.

Brookey, Robert Alan. *Reinventing the Male Homosexual: The Rhetoric and Power of the Gay Gene.* Bloomington: Indiana University Press, 2002.

Brown, Wendy. *Regulating Aversion: Tolerance in the Age of Identity and Empire.* Princeton, NJ: Princeton University Press, 2006.

Burke, Kenneth. *Language as Symbolic Action: Essays on Life, Literature, and Method.* Berkeley and Los Angeles: University of California Press, 1966.

———. *The Philosophy of Literary Form.* 1941. Berkeley and Los Angeles: University of California Press, 1973.

Burkett, Elinor. *The Gravest Show on Earth: America in the Age of AIDS.* Boston: Houghton Mifflin Company, 1995.

Butler, Judith. *Bodies That Matter: On the Discursive Limits of "Sex."* New York: Routledge, 1993.

——. *Excitable Speech: A Politics of the Performative.* New York: Routledge, 1997.

——. *Gender Trouble: Feminism and the Subversion of Identity.* New York: Routledge, 1999.

——. "Imitation and Gender Insubordination." In *Inside/Out: Lesbian Theories, Gay Theories,* ed. Diana Fuss, 13–31. New York: Routledge, 1991.

——. "Is Kinship Always Already Heterosexual?" *Differences: A Journal of Feminist Cultural Studies* 13 (2002): 14–44.

——. *The Psychic Life of Power: Theories in Subjection.* Stanford, CA: Stanford University Press, 1997.

——. *Undoing Gender.* New York: Routledge, 2004.

Carens, Joseph. *Culture, Citizenship, and Community: A Contextual Exploration of Justice as Evenhandedness.* New York: Oxford University Press, 2000.

Carson, Clayborne, and Shepard Carson. *A Call to Conscience: Landmark Speeches of Dr. Martin Luther King Jr.* New York: Warner Books, 2001.

Cohen, Cathy. *The Boundaries of Blackness: AIDS and the Breakdown of Black Politics.* Chicago: University of Chicago Press, 1999.

Condit, Celeste Michelle. "The Birth of Understanding: Chaste Science and the Harlot of the Arts." *Communication Monographs* 57 (1990): 323–327.

Condit, Celeste Michelle, and John Louis Lucaites. *Crafting Equality: America's Anglo-African Word.* Chicago: University of Chicago Press, 1993.

Corea, Gena. *The Invisible Epidemic: The Story of Women and AIDS.* New York: HarperCollins, 1992.

Crimp, Douglas. *AIDS: Cultural Analysis / Cultural Activism.* Cambridge, MA: MIT Press, 1988.

——. *AIDS Demographics.* Seattle: Bay Press, 1990.

——. *Melancholia and Moralism: Essays on AIDS and Queer Politics.* Cambridge, MA: MIT Press, 2002.

Cruikshank, Barbara. "Cultural Politics: Political Theory and the Foundations of Democratic Order." In *Cultural Studies and Political Theory,* ed. Jodi Dean, 63–79. Ithaca, NY: Cornell University Press, 2000.

Darsey, James. *The Prophetic Tradition and Radical Rhetoric in America.* New York: New York University Press, 1997.

de Certeau, Michel. *The Practice of Everyday Life.* Berkeley and Los Angeles: University of California Press, 1984.

Douglas, Mary. *Purity and Danger: An Analysis of the Concepts of Pollution and Taboo.* 1966. London: Routledge, 1996.

Dowsett, Gary. *Practicing Desire: Homosexual Sex in the Era of AIDS.* Stanford, CA: Stanford University Press, 1996.

Drescher, Jack. "I'm Your Handyman: A History of Reparative Therapies." *Journal of Homosexuality* 36 (1998): 19–42.

Duggan, Lisa. "Queering the State." In *Sex Wars: Sexual Dissent and Political Culture*, ed. Lisa Duggan and Nan Hunter, 178–193. New York: Routledge, 1995.

Duster, Troy. *Backdoor to Eugenics*. New York: Routledge, 1990.

Dyer, Richard. *Seven*. London: British Film Institute, 1999.

Edelman, Lee. *No Future: Queer Theory and the Death Drive*. Durham, NC: Duke University Press, 2004.

Ehlers, Nadine. "Hidden in Plain Sight: Defying Juridical Racialization in 'Rhinelander v. Rhinelander.'" *Communication and Critical/Cultural Studies* 1 (2004): 313–334.

Epstein, Steven. *Impure Science: AIDS, Activism, and the Politics of Knowledge*. Berkeley and Los Angeles: University of California Press, 1996.

Ewick, Patricia, and Susan S. Silbey. *The Common Place of Law: Stories from Everyday Life*. Chicago: University of Chicago Press, 1998.

Fausto-Sterling, Anne. "How to Build a Man." In *Constructing Masculinity*, ed. Maurice Berger, Brian Wallis, and Simon Watson, 127–134. New York: Routledge, 1995.

Florida Legislative Investigation Committee. "Homosexuality and Citizenship in Florida." Tallahassee, Florida, 1964.

Foucault, Michel. *Birth of the Clinic: An Archaeology of Medical Perception*. Trans. A. M. Sheridan Smith. 1973. New York: Vintage Books, 1994.

———. *Discipline and Punish: The Birth of the Prison*. Trans. Alan Sheridan. New York: Vintage Books, 1977.

———. *The History of Sexuality, Volume 1: An Introduction*. Trans. Robert Hurley. 1978. New York: Vintage Books, 1990.

———. *Power/Knowledge: Selected Interviews and Other Writings*. Ed. Colin Gordon. New York: Pantheon, 1980.

Fraser, Nancy. *Justice Interruptus: Critical Reflections on the 'Postsocialist' Condition*. New York: Routledge, 1996.

Ginsberg, Elaine. "The Politics of Passing." In *Passing and the Fictions of Identity*, ed. Elaine Ginsberg. Durham, NC: Duke University Press, 1996.

Gitlin, Todd. *The Twilight of Common Dreams: Why America Is Wracked by Culture Wars*. New York: Metropolitan Books, 1995.

Glied, Sherry. "The Circulation of Blood: AIDS, Blood, and the Economics of Information." In *Blood Feuds: AIDS, Blood, and the Politics of Medical Disaster*, ed. Eric Feldman and Ronald Bayer, 323–347. New York: Oxford University Press, 1999.

Goffman, Erving. *Stigma: Notes on the Management of Spoiled Identity*. 1963. New York: Simon and Schuster, 1986.

Gramsci, Antonio. *Selections from the Prison Notebooks*. Ed. Quintin Hoare and Geoffrey Nowell Smith. 1971. New York: International Publishers, 1999.

Grossberg, Lawrence. *We Gotta Get Out of This Place: Popular Conservatism and Postmodern Culture*. New York: Routledge, 1992.

Guttman, Amy, and Dennis Thompson. *Democracy and Disagreement*. Cambridge, MA: Harvard University Press, 1996.

Halberstam, Judith. *In a Queer Time and Place: Transgender Bodies, Subcultural Lives.* New York: New York University Press, 2005.

Hall, Stuart. "On Postmodernism and Articulation: An Interview with Stuart Hall." In *Stuart Hall: Critical Dialogues in Cultural Studies,* ed. David Morely and Kuan-Hsing Chen, 131–150. London: Routledge, 1996.

Halperin, David. *What Do Gay Men Want? An Essay on Sex, Risk, and Subjectivity.* Ann Arbor: University of Michigan Press, 2007.

Hamer, Dean, and Peter Copeland. *The Science of Desire: The Search for the Gay Gene and the Biology of Behavior.* New York: Simon and Schuster, 1994.

Hariman, Robert. "Prudence in the Twenty-first Century." In *Prudence: Classical Virtue, Postmodern Practice,* ed. Robert Hariman, 287–321. University Park: Pennsylvania State University Press, 2003.

Harvard Law Review. *Sexual Orientation and the Law.* Cambridge, MA: Harvard University Press, 1989.

Herek, Gregory M., Jared B. Jobe, and Ralph M. Carney, eds. *Out in Force: Sexual Orientation and the Military.* Chicago: University of Chicago Press, 1996.

Hewitt, Kim. *Mutilating the Body: Identity in Blood and Ink.* Bowling Green, OH: Bowling Green University Press, 1997.

Hochberg, Francine. "HIV/AIDS and Blood Donation Policies: A Comparative Study of Public Health Policies and Individual Rights Norms." *Duke Journal of Comparative and International Law* 12 (2002): 231–280.

Horner Jr., Donald H., and Michael T. Anderson. "Integration of Homosexuals into the Armed Forces: Racial and Gender Integration as a Point of Departure." In *Gays and Lesbians in the Military: Issues, Concerns, and Contrasts,* ed. Wilbur J. Scott and Sandra Carson Stanley, 247–260. New York: Aldine De Gruyter, 1994.

Institute of Medicine. *HIV and the Blood Supply: An Analysis of Crisis Decision Making.* Ed. Lauren Leveton, Harold C. Sox, and Michael Stoto. Washington, D.C.: National Academy Press, 1995.

Irons, Peter, and Stephanie Guitton. *May It Please the Court.* New York: New Press, 1993.

Ivie, Robert L. *Democracy and America's War on Terror.* Tuscaloosa: The University of Alabama Press, 2005.

Jeffreys, Sheila. "The Queer Disappearance of Lesbians: Sexuality in the Academy." *Women's Studies International Forum* 15 (1994): 249–472.

Johnson, E. Patrick. "'Quare' Studies, or (Almost) Everything I Know about Queer Studies I Learned from My Grandmother." *Text and Performance Quarterly* 21 (2001): 1–25.

Jones, James. *Bad Blood: The Tuskegee Syphilis Experiments.* New York: Free Press, 1981.

Joseph, May. *Nomadic Identities: The Performance of Citizenship.* Minneapolis: University of Minnesota Press, 1999.

Kaplan, Morris. *Sexual Justice: Democratic Citizenship and the Politics of Desire.* New York: Routledge, 1997.

Kauth, Michael R., and Dan Landis. "Applying Lessons Learned from Minority Integration in the Military." In *Out in Force: Sexual Orientation and the Military,* ed. Jared B. Jobe, Gregory M. Herek, and Ralph M. Carney, 86–105. Chicago: University of Chicago Press, 1996.

Kelley, Robin. "'We Are Not What We Seem': Rethinking Black Working-Class Opposition in the Jim Crow South." *Journal of American History* 80 (1993): 75–112.

Kelly, Joseph. "The Liability of Blood Banks and Manufacturers of Clotting Products to Recipients of HIV-Infected Blood: A Comparison of the Law and Reaction in the United States, Canada, Great Britain, Ireland, and Australia." *John Marshall Law Review* 27 (1994): 465–491.

Kirp, David. "The Politics of Blood: Hemophilia Activism in the AIDS Crisis." In *Blood Feuds: AIDS, Blood, and the Politics of Medical Disaster,* ed. Eric Feldman and Ronald Bayer, 293–321. New York: Oxford University Press, 1999.

Koegel, Paul. "Lessons Learned from the Experience of Domestic Police and Fire Departments." In *Out in Force: Sexual Orientation in the Military,* ed. Jared B. Jobe, Gregory M. Herek, and Ralph M. Carney, 131–153. Chicago: University of Chicago Press, 1996.

Kristeva, Julia. *Powers of Horror: An Essay on Abjection.* Trans. Leon Roudiez. New York: Columbia University Press, 1982.

———. *Strangers to Ourselves.* Trans. Leon Roudiez. New York: Columbia University Press, 1991.

Kymlicka, Will. *Multicultural Citizenship: A Liberal Theory of Minority Rights.* New York: Oxford University Press, 1996.

Lahiri, Shompa. "Performing Identity: Colonial Migrants, Passing, and Mimicry between the Wars." *Cultural Geographies* 10 (2003): 408–423.

Lemire, Elise Virginia. *"Miscegenation": Making Race in America.* Philadelphia: University of Pennsylvania Press, 2002.

Lévi-Strauss, Claude. *The Elementary Structures of Kinship.* Boston: Beacon Press, 1969.

Lipsitz, George. *Time Passages: Collective Memory and American Popular Culture.* Minneapolis: University of Minnesota Press, 1990.

Lister, Ruth. *Citizenship: Feminist Perspectives.* New York: New York University Press, 1997.

Love, Spencie. *One Blood: The Death and Resurrection of Charles R. Drew.* Chapel Hill: University of North Carolina Press, 1996.

Lyne, John, and Henry Howe. "Punctuated Equilibria: Rhetorical Dynamics of a Scientific Controversy." *Quarterly Journal of Speech* 72 (1986): 132–147.

Maistrellis, Christina. "American Red Cross v. S.G. & A.E.: An Open Door to the Federal Courts for Federally Chartered Corporations." *Emory Law Journal* 45 (1996): 771–804.

Mann, Michael. "Has Globalization Ended the Rise of the Nation-State?" In *The Global Transformations Reader: An Introduction to the Globalization Debate,* ed. David Held and Anthony McGrew, 136–147. Cambridge, MA: Polity Press, 2000.

Martin, Emily. "The Egg and the Sperm: How Science Has Constructed a Romance

Based on Stereotypical Male-Female Roles." *Signs: Journal of Women in Culture and Society* 16 (1991): 485–501.

——. *Flexible Bodies: Tracking Immunity in American Culture from the Days of Polio to the Age of AIDS.* Boston: Beacon Press, 1994.

Marvin, Carolyn, and David W. Ingle. *Blood Sacrifice and the Nation: Totem Rituals and the American Flag.* Cambridge: Cambridge University Press, 1999.

McDorman, Todd. "Controlling Death: Bio-Power and the Right-to-Die Controversy." *Communication and Critical/Cultural Studies* 2 (2005): 257–279.

Michaels, Walter Benn. *The Trouble with Diversity: How We Learned to Love Identity and Ignore Inequality.* New York: Metropolitan Books, 2006.

Miller, Toby. *Cultural Citizenship: Cosmopolitanism, Consumerism, and Television in a Neoliberal Age.* Philadelphia: Temple University Press, 2007.

Moore, Patrick. *Beyond Shame: Reclaiming the Abandoned History of Radical Gay Sexuality.* Boston: Beacon Press, 2004.

Morris III, Charles E. "Pink Herring and the Fourth Persona: J. Edgar Hoover's Sex Crime Panic." *Quarterly Journal of Speech* 88 (2002): 228–244.

——. "'The Responsibility of the Critic': F. O. Matthiessen's Homosexual Palimpsest." *Quarterly Journal of Speech* 84 (1998): 261–282.

Morrow, Rona. "AIDS and Immigration: The United States Attempts to Deport a Disease." In *AIDS Law and Policy,* ed. Arthur S. Leonard, 278–282. Houston, TX: John Marshall Publishing Company, 1995.

Mosse, George. *Nationalism and Sexuality: Respectability and Abnormal Sexuality in Modern Europe.* New York: Howard Fertig, 1985.

Mouffe, Chantal. *The Democratic Paradox.* London: Verso, 2000.

——. *The Return of the Political.* London: Verso, 1993.

Murray, Thomas. "The Poisoned Gift: AIDS and Blood." In *A Disease of Society: Cultural and Institutional Response to AIDS,* ed. David P. Willis, Dorothy Nelkin, and Scott V. Parris, 216–240. Cambridge: Cambridge University Press, 1991.

National Defense Research Institute (U.S.). *Sexual Orientation and U.S. Military Personnel Policy: Options and Assessment.* Santa Monica, CA: Rand, 1993.

Nelkin, Dorothy. "Cultural Perspectives on Blood." In *Blood Feuds: AIDS, Blood, and the Politics of Medical Disaster,* ed. Eric Feldman and Ronald Bayer, 273–292. New York: Oxford University Press, 1999.

Nelson, John S. "Prudence as Republican Politics in American Popular Culture." In *Prudence: Classical Virtue, Postmodern Practice,* ed. Robert Hariman, 229–257. University Park: Pennsylvania State University Press, 2003.

Noakes, Jeremy, and Geoffrey Pridham. *Documents of Nazism, 1919–1945.* London: Jonathan Cape, 1974.

Oravec, Christine L. "Fanny Wright and the Enforcing of Prudence: Women, Propriety, and Transgression in Nineteenth-Century Public Oratory of the United States." In *Prudence: Classical Virtue, Postmodern Practice,* ed. Robert Hariman, 189–225. University Park: Pennsylvania State University Press, 2003.

Patton, Cindy. *Fatal Advice: How Safe-Sex Education Went Wrong.* Durham, NC: Duke University Press, 1996.

——. "From Nation to Family: Containing African AIDS." In *The Gender/Sexuality Reader: Culture, History, Political Economy,* ed. Roger N. Lancaster and Micaela di Leonardo, 279–290. New York: Routledge, 1997.

——. *Globalizing AIDS.* Minneapolis: University of Minnesota Press, 2002.

——. *Inventing AIDS.* New York: Routledge, 1990.

——. *Sex and Germs: The Politics of AIDS.* Boston: South End Press, 1985.

——. "Tremble, Hetero Swine!" In *Fear of a Queer Planet: Queer Politics and Social Theory,* ed. Michael Warner, 143–177. Minneapolis: University of Minnesota Press, 1993.

Perl, Gisella. *I Was a Doctor in Auschwitz.* New York: International Universities Press, 1948.

Pezzullo, Phaedra. "Resisting 'National Breast Cancer Awareness Month': The Rhetoric of Counterpublics and Their Cultural Performances." *Quarterly Journal of Speech* 89 (2003): 345–365.

Phelan, Peggy. *Unmarked: The Politics of Performance.* London: Routledge, 1993.

Pieplow, Kathryn. "AIDS, Blood Banks and the Court: The Legal Response to Transfusion-Acquired Disease." *South Dakota Law Review* 38 (1993): 609–640.

Piliavin, Jane Allyn, and Peter L. Callero. *Giving Blood: The Development of an Altruistic Identity.* Baltimore, MD: Johns Hopkins University Press, 1991.

Plummer, Ken. *Intimate Citizenship: Private Decision and Public Dialogues.* Seattle: University of Washington Press, 2003.

——. *Telling Sexual Stories: Power, Change, and Social Worlds.* London: Routledge, 1995.

Pocock, J.G.A. "The Ideal of Citizenship since Classical Times." *Queen's Quarterly* 99 (1992): 33–55.

Ports, Suki. "Needed (for Women and Children)." In *AIDS: Cultural Analysis/Cultural Activism,* ed. Douglas Crimp, 169–176. Cambridge, MA: MIT Press, 1988.

Prelli, Lawrence. "Rhetorical Logic and the Integration of Rhetoric and Science." *Communication Monographs* 57 (1990): 315–322.

Proctor, Robert. *Racial Hygiene: Medicine under the Nazis.* Cambridge, MA: Harvard University Press, 1988.

Red Gold: The Epic Story of Blood. Dir. Nick Read. Films for the Humanities and Sciences, 2002. Videocassette.

Reeves, Carol. "Rhetoric and the AIDS Virus Hunt." *Quarterly Journal of Speech* 84 (1998): 1–22.

Rigg, Bryan Mark. *Hitler's Jewish Soldiers: The Untold Story of Nazi Racial Laws and Men of Jewish Descent in the German Military.* Lawrence: University Press of Kansas, 2002.

Robinson, Amy. "It Takes One to Know One: Passing and Communities of Common Interest." *Critical Inquiry* 20 (1994): 715–736.

Rousseau, Jean-Jacques. "Discourse on Political Economy." In *Rousseau's Political Writ-*

ings, ed. Alan Ritter and Julia Conaway Bondanella. New York: W. W. Norton, 1988.

Schneider, David. *American Kinship: A Cultural Account.* Chicago: University of Chicago Press, 1980.

———. "Kinship, Nationality, and Religion in American Culture: Towards a Definition of Kinship." In *Symbolic Anthropology: A Reader in the Study of Symbols and Meanings,* ed. Janet Dolgin, David Kemnitzer, and David Schneider, 63–71. New York: Columbia University Press, 1977.

Scott, James C. *Domination and the Arts of Resistance: Hidden Transcripts.* New Haven, CT: Yale University Press, 1990.

———. *Seeing Like a State: How Certain Schemes to Improve the Human Condition Have Failed.* New Haven, CT: Yale University Press, 1998.

Scott, Wilbur, and Sandra Carson Stanley, eds. *Gays and Lesbians in the Military: Issues, Concerns, and Contrasts.* New York: Aldine de Gruyter, 1994.

Sedgwick, Eve Kosofsky. *Epistemology of the Closet.* Berkeley and Los Angeles: University of California Press, 1990.

———. "Queer Performativity: Henry James's *The Art of the Novel.*" *GLQ* 1 (1993): 1–16.

Shilts, Randy. *And the Band Played On: Politics, People, and the AIDS Epidemic.* New York: St. Martin's Press, 1987.

Shugart, Helene. "Performing Ambiguity: The Passing of Ellen Degeneres." *Text and Performance Quarterly* 23 (2003): 30–54.

Slack, Jennifer Daryl. "The Theory and Method of Articulation in Cultural Studies." In *Stuart Hall: Critical Dialogues in Cultural Studies,* ed. David Morely and Kuan-Hsing Chen, 112–127. London: Routledge, 1996.

Slagle, R. Anthony. "In Defense of Queer Nation: From Identity Politics to a Politics of Difference." *Western Journal of Communication* 59 (1995): 85–102.

Sloop, John M. *Disciplining Gender: Rhetorics of Sex Identity in Contemporary U.S. Culture.* Amherst: University of Massachusetts Press, 2004.

———. "Disciplining the Transgendered: Brandon Teena, Public Representation, and Normativity." *Western Journal of Communication* 64 (2000): 165–189.

Smith, Barbara Herrnstein. *Scandalous Knowledge: Science, Truth, and the Human.* Durham, NC: Duke University Press, 2005.

Spradlin, Anna. "The Price of 'Passing': A Lesbian Perspective on Authenticity in Organizations." *Management Communication Quarterly* 11 (1998): 598–605.

Squires, Catherine, and Daniel Brouwer. "In/Discernible Bodies: The Politics of Passing in Dominant and Marginal Media." *Critical Studies in Media Communication* 19 (2002): 283–310.

Starr, Douglas. *Blood: An Epic History of Medicine and Commerce.* New York: Alfred Knopf, 1998.

Stoler, Ann Laura. *Race and the Education of Desire: Foucault's History of Sexuality and the Colonial Order of Things.* Durham, NC: Duke University Press, 1995.

Sturken, Marita. *Tangled Memories: The Vietnam War, the AIDS Epidemic, and the Politics of Remembering*. Berkeley and Los Angeles: University of California Press, 1997.

Summerrise, Reginald, and Pamela DeCarlo. *What Are Heterosexual Men's HIV Prevention Needs?* Center for AIDS Prevention Studies at the University of California, San Francisco, 2001.

Taylor, Diana. *The Archive and the Repertoire: Performing Cultural Memory in the Americas*. Durham, NC: Duke University Press, 2003.

Titmuss, Richard. *The Gift Relationship: From Human Blood to Social Policy*. London: George Allen & Unwin Ltd., 1970.

Triechler, Paula. *How to Have Theory in an Epidemic: Cultural Chronicles of AIDS*. Durham, NC: Duke University Press, 1999.

Tropiano, Stephen. *The Prime Time Closet: A History of Gays and Lesbians on TV*. New York: Applause Theatre and Cinema Books, 2002.

U.S. Army Medical Service. *Blood Program in World War II*. Washington, D.C.: Office of the Surgeon General, Department of the Army, 1964.

U.S. Food and Drug Administration. *FDA Workshop on Behavior-Based Donor Deferrals in the NAT Era*. March 8, 2006.

Vaid, Urvashi. *Virtual Equality: The Mainstreaming of Gay and Lesbian Liberation*. New York: Anchor Books, 1995.

Warner, Michael. *Fear of a Queer Planet: Queer Politics and Social Theory*. Minneapolis: University of Minnesota Press, 1993.

———. *Publics and Counterpublics*. New York: Zone Books, 2002.

———. *The Trouble with Normal: Sex, Politics, and the Ethics of Queer Life*. New York: Free Press, 1999.

Watney, Simon. *Policing Desire: Pornography, AIDS, and the Media*. Minneapolis: University of Minnesota Press, 1987.

Weeks, Jeffrey. *Invented Moralities: Sexual Values in an Age of Uncertainty*. New York: Columbia University Press, 1995.

Weston, Kath. "Do Clothes Make the Woman? Gender, Performance Theory, and Lesbian Eroticism." *Genders* 17 (1993): 1–21.

Wiegman, Robyn. *American Anatomies: Theorizing Race and Gender*. Durham, NC: Duke University Press, 1995.

Yingling, Thomas. *AIDS and the National Body*. Durham, NC: Duke University Press, 1997.

Young, Iris Marion. "Abjection and Oppression: Dynamics of Unconscious Racism, Sexism, and Homophobia." In *Crises in Continental Philosophy*, ed. Charles Scott, Arleen Dallery, and P. Holley Roberts, 201–213. Albany: State University of New York Press, 1990.

———. *Inclusion and Democracy*. New York: Oxford University Press, 2000.

———. *Intersecting Voices: Dilemmas of Gender, Political Philosophy, and Policy*. Princeton, NJ: Princeton University Press, 1997.

Zelizer, Barbie. "Reading the Past against the Grain: The Shape of Memory Studies." *Critical Studies in Mass Communication* 12 (1995): 214–239.

Index